KEEP SMILING

Keep Smiling
Jack Saroyan, D.D.S.

Library of Congress Control Number: 2025908271

Published by Spines
ISBN 979-8-89950-549-2

Spines

KEEP SMILING

AN INSIDER'S LOOK AT DENTAL CARE

DR. JACK M. SAROYAN, D.D.S., F.A.G.D., F.A.C.D.

CONTENTS

In memory of my parents Meran Manoog Saroyan
and Alice Samarjian Hagopian Saroyan
(who were) Genocide Survivors

FOREWORD

Teeth have always meant far more than we have bothered to put forward in a convenient form. The last time I visited my cousin Jack Saroyan in his office on Sutter Street in San Francisco, I urged him to gather into an enormous book the entire lore and science of teeth—which, of course, would have to include a history of dentistry, which, not so long ago, included the giving of a haircut to a customer and even the use of a few leaches in a theory of tonic value. I hope that Jack does that, but if he doesn't, I hope as editor of the California Dental Association Journal—a magazine that I find fascinating—he puts the program or assignment, or job before a committee, so that perhaps a dozen dentists may do this job.

This excerpt is taken from an article entitled "About Teeth and Dentists", in the CDA Journal, December 1976, by author and playwright, William Saroyan.

INTRODUCTION

The practice of dentistry has been much more than a livelihood for me. Dentistry has been a true calling. I have a passion for my profession—one that has shaped me and that I have worked to shape as well. In this introduction, I would like to share with you the depth and breadth of my dental experiences, so you can feel confident reading this book and learning from me.

I have influenced my profession through private dental practice, involvement in professional governance at various levels, and teaching experience. The foundation of my profession, the prevention of disease, has been present from the early history of civilization. In 335 BC, the Greek philosopher Aristotle associated dental cavities with sweet foods, such as figs. Avoiding sweet foods is a strategy for cavity prevention.

I have been shaped by my profession and have come to embrace the concept of prevention in my family life and lifestyle. For example, after the 1989 earthquake in San Francisco, I immediately fortified my home to prevent future damage. (This was even before the government recommended residents to do so.) I wanted to have a house that was stronger than when its original construction. Seat belts were installed in a 1956 Dodge to reduce the risk of injury during car accidents, and a 1964 Volvo was equipped with three-point seat belts before they became mandatory in California. Fortunately, although I always strapped on the belt, I never needed the seat belt restraints.

I have participated in local, state, and national dental organizations. I am a life member of the American Dental Association (ADA), the California Dental Association (CDA), and the San Francisco Dental Society (SFDS).

After graduating from dental school, I served two years active duty as a dental officer and six years in the US Navy Dental Corps Reserves. Upon returning home to San Francisco, I worked for my family dentist for one year and then opened my own office.

I received two honorary fellowship degrees: One is as a Fellow of the Academy of General Dentistry (FAGD) to recognize that I had completed additional courses beyond the legal requirement for dentists. The other is as a Fellow of the American College of Dentists (FACD). Only 4 percent of American dentists have been eligible for this distinction. Nominees must be outstanding in one or more of their contributions to community affairs, professional governance, dental education, research, or publications to earn this fellowship degree.

These degrees were earned through careful review and screening processes. One or two organizational members confidentially nominate someone for a fellowship degree (and the accompanying membership to the organization). Then the local members in the region are consulted as to the worthiness of the nominee. If the local members agree that the nominee is outstanding in all respects, the nominee is then eligible for membership.

During my full-time practice career, I always made time to be active in the governance of the various levels of organized dentistry. I served as secretary, editor, and later, president of the San Francisco Dental Society (SFDS).

On becoming editor of the Journal of the California Dental Association, the CDA sent me to an ADA-sponsored dental editor's seminar in Columbus, Ohio, conducted by the School of Journalism at Ohio State University. It was a week of intensive training, with nightly seminars in addition to lectures and writing daily. A critique of my first edited CDA journal was done by the course instructors. Later, I was also trained to be a spokesperson for the CDA as well.

I was recognized by the ADA for my humanitarian dental services to the children, seminarians, and military cadets in the Republic of Armenia. I made five trips, for two weeks each, with several other Californian Armenian American dentists, done at our own expense and donations from dentists and family, except for one grant of three thousand dollars from the University of the Pacific. I saw and treated large dental cavities of the children and received the appreciation of parents and village people. I returned twice a year afterward to introduce and attempt to implement fluoridated table salt for the prevention of cavities. I knew that our treatment was dentally, medically, and morally beneficial, but we were just scratching the surface of a huge problem that the government was sweeping under the rug.

What was needed was the availability of table salt that is fluoridated because water fluoridation was not economically possible. The fluoridated table salt could easily be manufactured in Armenia because Armenia has a salt mine and already produces its own salt. I had several meetings with the head of the salt company. I even brought a salt engineer to Armenia at my own expense to inspect the salt plant for its ability to make fluoridated salt. He found the plant in good condition and that the special equipment needed could be easily installed. I had even more discussions with the various ministers of health over an eight-year period, returning twice a year for them to approve any changes.

We came close to implementation, but they were not trained on the benefits of prevention of disease, nor were they motivated—even though the efficacy and use of iodized and fluoridated salt containing sodium fluoride was being used in Belarus, an adjacent former Soviet nation. Returning home from the Republic of Armenia, I realized that we dentists here in America were not doing enough to prevent cavities and gum diseases at home. This was an awakening for me to author this book. We need to improve the dental health of our children and young adults by both types of fluoridation, water and table salt.

My interests in volunteer teaching came from the example of the dental instructors I had at school. As a dental student, most of my instructors were practicing dentists who volunteered their time to teach on the adjunct faculty at the College of Physicians and Surgeons, which later became the University of the Pacific (UOP), Dugoni School of Dentistry. This private dental school has no state or federal funding and depends on the student tuition and income from the clinic to survive. I admired my teaching dentist instructors who were not salaried; they inspired me to want to be like them when I graduated. I have volunteered on a pro bono basis as well and have served for the past twenty-three years. I have given back with my talent, time, and treasure to the school because I felt indebted for the education I received.

At first, I was asked to teach some laboratory courses, then I was assigned to the clinic floor with the patients. Then I was asked to help teach a dental ethics course after serving on the state dental board. I continue to contribute, giving annual lectures on three subjects: dental history, salt fluoridation, and how to teach flossing—all of which are not covered in the regular curriculum. Students should be familiar with these subjects.

Recently at an alumni meeting, I was awarded the Medallion of Distinction. This is the highest honor that a graduate can receive for contributions of service to dental education, the profession, and the local and international communities. It was truly a humble experience with an audience numbering several hundred people. My family was also present. After the dean placed a ribbon bearing the medal around my neck, I was asked to speak. After thanking everyone who helped me become a dentist, I said that I wished my parents could have witnessed this high honor because they had made significant financial sacrifices to support my nine years of college education when student education loans were not available. I introduced my children, son-in-law, and especially, my wife, who not only supported me, but took an active role in the dental school's Women's Auxiliary as their president. We are a dental family, through and through.

For several years I served in the House of Delegates for both the ADA and the CDA; these bodies govern dentists' professional activities. But my most rewarding and challenging position, while in dental practice, was to serve on the California State Board of Dental Examiners. I helped "wash the profession's dirty linen," as the saying goes, and oversaw the examination of thousands of applicants. The year I was president I got writer's cramps signing over 1,500 dental licenses! Moreover, my experience overseeing what constituted malpractice and substandard dental care made me realize that regulations alone do not protect the public. I learned that unless your dentist is taught to have and develops a sense of ethical practices, you may not receive the best of care. A trusting relationship between an ethical doctor and the patient is necessary for the best care.

To serve on the state board, I had to study and learn all about the regulations of the California Dental Practice Act. Part of our responsibility was to examine and qualify dentists to practice in California, which included the dentists who came from out of state. We had the power to remove a dentist's license to practice. Imagine having your ability to make a living taken away from you. What becomes of your family? How would you pay the home mortgage expenses or purchase the local groceries? Of course, this extreme decision to revoke a license was infrequent and unusual. Unless the person committed a criminal act or refused to sign a waiver of rights to continue practicing with our supervision. We could subject a wrongdoer to several years of periodic reporting and quarterly inspections. We could require more continuing education courses for dentists, allowing them to continue their practices under certain additional stipulations or conditions.

I was appointed to the state board by California's Governor George Deukmejian. Only six dentists were appointed to serve along with a few lay people. By the time I was appointed to the board, the governor and I had known each other for years. We first met when he was a state senator representing Long Beach. When he ran for attorney general, I was a campaign co-chairman in San Francisco. When he decided to run for governor, I helped him with his political campaign.

The California state legislature determines board member salaries, which are funded from licensure fees paid by the dentists and dental hygienists. But board members do not do it for the pay: Time out of the office was more costly for me than the payment given to me by the legislature. I remained on the board for nine years and became president for one year. As heady and powerful as that may be, I spent at least fifty days out of my office going to board meetings and conducting examinations annually.

For me, the most uncomfortable aspect of my board duty was conducting the dental hygiene examination. By this time, the dental hygienists were conducting the dental hygienists' examinations, but they needed a board dentist to supervise the exams. I volunteered to attend and supervise since I was close to the dental hygiene school at the University of California in San Francisco. Little did I know what this job was going to entail.

The chair of the dental hygienists would introduce me to the candidates at the beginning of the examination. Later on, I was asked to inform a candidate that they did not finish on time or that they did not pass the exam—and therefore failed the examination.

The chair of the dental hygienists would give me the seat number of the failing candidate after the morning examination and again after the afternoon examination. I went to that student to deliver the bad news. Every young lady—in these years, the students were all women—burst into tears. After my first experience, I started taking Kleenex tissues with me. I now teach freshmen students at UOP Dental School in San Francisco, to examine, diagnose, and treat gum diseases.

Between my dental practice years and my retirement years from active dental practice, I have served the adjunct faculty of the UOP dental school for twenty-three years. I enjoy helping the future generation of dentists. I want them to always place their patient's interests ahead of their own interests. Over these years, I still like teaching first-year students because they are the most impressionable and receptive students.

Now that you know the extent of my experience and my passion for dentistry, you can trust that I know what I'm talking about when I raise all the issues we will cover in the rest of this book.

In the first chapter, I'll explain how your dental health impacts your general health and vice versa. Understanding this important concept can motivate you to keep up with good oral hygiene habits.

In chapter 2, Prevention vs. Treatment, I will go over the value of preventing dental problems beyond treating them. And I will explain to you how prevention does not stop at treatment. You will learn why preventive measures benefit your health and save you money.

In chapter 3, although the benefits of fluoride have been known for the past 79 years, there is still controversy about community water fluoridation. You will learn how fluoride was discovered to help in the prevention of cavities, how it works, and what are its limitations. We'll look at the various challenges to fluoridated water supply, from community resistance to its expense and the maintenance of facilities. And we will outline where fluoridated water is possible, and where it cannot be supplied. Finally, I will share with you a good option for providing fluoride where fluoridated water is not possible: fluoridated table salt. And we will discuss the benefits, and resistance, to that option too.

In chapter 4 about Dental Education, I will explain the training of dental students to become physicians of the mouth. And how your dentist is also trained to detect medical problems such as diabetes and oral cancer. But in doing so, I also cover how schools neglect some of the basic preventive practices of maintaining good oral health.

In the fifth chapter on Dental Insurance Plans, I will discuss how this popular employee benefit has attracted many more people to seek dental care. But how this insurance is really a form of prepaid dental care and what the resulting implications mean to patients.

In chapter 6 on Subsidized Dental Clinics for Children and Adults, I will identify all the options in your community to find dental clinics that are more affordable than private dental offices. At the same time, I will talk about some of their shortcomings of providing personal dental care.

In chapter 7 about The Rise of Corporate Dentistry, I will tell you about this new kind of dental service model that is growing. And what some dentists say is the commercialization of the dental profession.

With chapter 8 about the History and a Discussion of Dental Care versus Medical Care, I discuss the fragmentation of the healing arts professions that occurred many years ago, but still unequally influence health today. Many of my patients with Medicare benefits have always wondered why dental care is not provided under this program for seniors. Here ae some answers to that question.

In chapter 9 on Cosmetic Dentistry, I discuss all the options besides tooth bleaching, which the public has embraced. Americans want beautifully straight and even teeth to smile with, talk with, sing with and eat with for all their life long. And the American dental profession is ready and willing to deliver what they deserve and want. But shouldn't the health of your teeth and gums be treated first? Of course!

In this chapter on Dental Specialties, I review all the different kinds of dental specialists who are available for dental care beyond the general practice dentist care. Upon researching this subject, I was even surprised at what has evolved in new specialties. Why your dentist may refer you to a specialist is talked about. Think of your general dentist as "the Jack of all specialties (trades), but master of none."

In chapter 11 with the title For Dentists Only, I talk directly to my fellow dentists who want to serve their patients better by teaching them how to train their patients to floss better. Of course, Dear Reader, you may wish to read what I have to say too.

Chapter 12 on How to Brush and Floss properly is a detailed step-by-step account of self-training to floss effectively. Just as learning how to type on a keyboard does not come naturally, neither does flossing your teeth. Among all personal hygiene tasks, flossing one's teeth can be particularly challenging.

The concluding chapter 13 Conclusion, Advice and Thought on the Future, sums it all up.

Now, let's dive in, so you learn why healthy teeth and gums matter to maintaining your general health—and you can get started actively keeping your mouth and body healthy. You can begin your reading with chapter 1, or feel free to go to whatever chapter you have a particular interest in reading first. You will get an insider's look at dentistry, and I sincerely hope it will inspire you to keep smiling!

1

THE IMPORTANCE OF DENTAL HEALTH

I remember a few years ago hearing about a teenage boy who'd made national TV news because of a horrific outcome due to an untreated infected tooth. He was on a dental Medicaid welfare insurance plan in New York, and his mother took him to the dental clinic. However, there was some delay in having the tooth removed. The infection became worse, and he needed to be hospitalized. The infection had persisted so long that he got blood poisoning and died in the hospital. How tragic that a child died for lack of the immediate dental treatment of an infected tooth.

This example of the seriousness of an infected tooth can happen to anyone when no emergency dental care is available or if the treatment of dental abscess or cellulitis is delayed. This chapter will show various dental problems and treatment that are related to your general health. The relationship of our dental health cannot be separated from our medical wellbeing.

Sometimes doing root canal treatment to save an infected tooth can result in the patient ending up in the hospital. As a young, inexperienced navy dentist, I was assigned by the senior dentist to take care of a sailor who was in pain with an abscessed upper right canine tooth. I first got him out of pain by numbing the tooth and told him I could save his tooth with root canal treatment. The X-ray showed me that the infection was only at the tip of the root, and the gum and bone were healthy. Now remember, I was relatively new to my profession. I had just graduated dental school eight months earlier, and in dental school I had only successfully treated three infected teeth with root canal treatments. The young sailor agreed to the treatment. Having his consent, I made the tooth numb and went ahead with removing the infected nerve, then cleaning and irrigating the root canal. I temporarily sealed the tooth and sent him back to work with an appointment to complete the treatment the following week.

He came back two days later with his right face so swollen that it almost closed his right eye. I called over to the senior dental captain, and he decided that I should take the patient—in my car—to the naval hospital several miles away to see an oral surgeon immediately. I agreed wholeheartedly. When we got there, I explained my treatment to the oral surgeon, and he agreed to take over the treatment. After several days in the hospital, on a potent intravenous antibiotic, the swelling began to subside, and the patient returned to me about two weeks later. Meanwhile, I discussed with my captain why my treatment had gone wrong. He told me that sometimes it is better to allow the tooth to self-drain before sealing it. Fortunately, when the patient was better, I continued the treatment and saved the tooth. It was a lesson that I will never forget.

An infected upper front tooth can cause injury to the eye nerve or it could continue to the brain. An untreated lower tooth infection can descend into the neck or lungs. Our tooth roots are so close to our vital organs, such as the eyes, brain, and lungs, and the health of these organs is critical to our overall health.

Each tooth, itself, is an organ, composed of different types of tissue that perform a function. Each one of our twenty teeth during childhood and each of our thirty-two teeth during adulthood can become infected and cause serious health problems if not treated. These tooth organs in our mouth, which are surrounded by our gums and a specialized type of bone, must be cared for and be free of disease for good general health throughout our lifetime. It should be no wonder that the health of our teeth and gums can influence or be linked to systemic medical conditions. The medical profession now recognizes that inflammation of the gums is a contributory factor in several medical diseases. The correlation between low infant birth weight with expectant mothers experiencing gingivitis or periodontitis during pregnancy was first observed in scientific studies. These underweight infants or premature babies, called preemies, are common in the United States and are treated in special sections of the hospital. We have pediatric neonatal specialists and nurses who care for them until they are able to be returned to their mother. However, in countries that do not have the essential specialized equipment and specialists with neonatal training, these infants do not survive.

Although I have treated many pregnant patients, I have never investigated or followed up on the condition of their newborn infants. However, gum or periodontal research has shown, since 1996, that the toxic chemicals of inflamed gum tissues can easily enter the bloodstream and affect the fetus and the mother. To give you a sense of the size of your gum tissues, imagine this: if your gum tissue was all spread out, it would be about the size of the palm of your hand. Imagine a part of your skin that had a similar size infection; now you can realize how the mother and infant would be so adversely affected.

Inflammation anywhere in the body is harmful to our general health, whether it arises from the gums or another area of the body. Inflammation spreads by way of the lymph nodes and blood vessels of the cardiovascular system, which includes the arteries and veins. Studies have proven the connection between heart health and dental health, and it's worth understanding that further. For instance, the thickening of the artery wall in response to inflammation reduces and restricts the space inside the vessel (in the lumen). This condition results in raising blood pressure, which is a medical condition called hypertension, prevalent among our aging population. This condition can be monitored easily in the office or at home by using a portable blood pressure cuff that is sold at all drug stores. Dental students at UOP are trained to record blood pressure along with other vital signs during a dental examination. Your dentist may refer you for medical care if you have high blood pressure. Hypertension is the precursor of stroke which is an attack of the brain. Periodontitis, which means inflammation of the gums, increases the risk of a transient ischemic attack (TIA), sometimes called a ministroke. Often, minor stroke events can lead to more severe strokes that may result in permanent speech impairment or limb paralysis.

As early as the 1970s cardiac surgeons discovered P. gingivalis in the diseased heart valves. This microbe is the most virulent bacteria of periodontitis, and of other bacteria related to gum diseases. Endocarditis is defined as a bacterial attack on the interior of the heart which usually affects the heart valves first. It is now recognized that patients diagnosed with endocarditis have twice the likelihood of developing periodontal disease. Today, cardiac surgeons and some cardiologists require dental checkups to assure them that the gums are healthy and not inflamed before performing heart surgery or noninvasive vascular procedures.

Periodontitis and diabetes are thought to connect dental diseases with medical conditions directly. These diseases exhibit a reciprocal relationship. In other words, diabetes increases the risk for periodontitis, and periodontal inflammation increases the risk of diabetes. The susceptibility to periodontitis is increased by about threefold in people with diabetes. Furthermore, when I read the research on the various medical diseases that can occur with underlying periodontitis, I learned that the risk of cardiorenal (heart and kidney) disease is three times higher in diabetic people with severe periodontitis than diabetic people without severe periodontitis. Oral and periodontal health should be promoted as integral components of diabetes management.

To emphasize the prevalence and importance of diabetes in caring for our dental patients, every new patient at UOP is evaluated for diabetes along with recording other vital signs, such as blood pressure, pulse, and breathing rate. In this manner the students can often identify prediabetic patients and refer them for early medical care. A handheld device and a finger prick blood sample are used to evaluate glucose levels in-office. For diabetic patients, this test is conducted at each appointment to verify their health status and suitability for treatment.

Another set of organs that are affected by bacterial inflammation of the gums is our lungs. As we breathe through our nose and mouth, the bacteria and inflammation of advanced periodontal disease can also affect the bronchial tubes and our lungs.

We all have dormant or inactive pneumonia bacteria in our lung tissue lining. When resistance is low or the immune system response is weakened by periodontal disease, this condition can lead to pneumonia, which is a leading cause of death among the elderly. Here again, preventive dental checkups could alert your dentist to recommend a referral to your medical doctor.

Oral and colorectal cancers are also risks of periodontal disease. Oral cancer has a high morbidity rate because it is often detected late and can spread to vital organs in the throat and neck. Most physicians do not normally do this examination. I do not know what their training is, but I do know that all dentists have this training and do this cancer screening examination of mouth tissues at least annually. Another benefit of periodic dental examinations, besides monitoring your dental health of your teeth and gums, is this oral cancer screening.

Recent research has established a connection between gum disease and Alzheimer's disease. This condition was identified through brain scans conducted on patients experiencing cognitive issues. The early signs of the alkaloid deposits that identify this disease are higher in patients with periodontal disease. Here again, the source of infection can arise from the condition of long-standing gingivitis or periodontitis. This bacterial infection can permeate the blood-brain barrier to cause or worsen this mental disease.

Dentists can distinguish between periodontitis and halitosis. Bad breath is not just a small or silly problem for people going to a job interview or on a first date. Part of my new patient examination is to smell my new patients' breath. Most of the time, my patient's breath is sweet smelling and not offensive. I then assure them, even though they may not have asked me if their breath is fresh. After all, bad breath is a social taboo that no one wants to have, yet people can be unaware of having it.

We have all smelled someone's breath that has a fetid odor. I have had patients whose wives or girlfriends sent them to me because they had bad breath. But there are several varied reasons and conditions that can result in bad breath. Although, if it is constantly the same fetid odor, it is more than likely due to gum infection; or they may not be cleaning their teeth or tongue thoroughly. I have detected patients with prediabetic, acetone breath and referred them to a medical doctor for a glucose tolerance test. Some older patients who take multiple medications may develop xerostomia (dry mouth), which can lead to halitosis. Or if they have removable dentures that are not cleaned properly, this is another reason for bad breath.

Of course, if you eat a lot of garlic, we all know that it can affect your breath. Certain other foods and drinks, like onions, fish, sardines, and alcohol, can affect your breath for hours. Breath odors can also arise from gastric (stomach) upset or more serious problems like stomach cancer. Just being extremely nervous or upset about a matter can affect your breath. Ninety percent of the time, halitosis arises from dental conditions of the teeth, gums, or tongue and is preventable. Rarely, halitosis can come from one of many different medical conditions, such as disorders in the head sinuses, nasal cavity, throat, esophagus, lungs, stomach, liver, kidney and pancreas.

I will never forget a dentist whom I once went to as a patient before dentists wore masks and gloves. He smoked so much that his breath and fingers wreaked of tobacco odor. The smell was an awful experience for me, but a good lesson to learn. When I became a dental student, I smoked. I made sure that my bad habit did not offend any of my patients. I would not smoke in the dental clinic or office and limited my smoking to after meals and weekends. Later, my wife helped me quit smoking; she felt that a health professional should have ideal health habits and should be an example to their patients. I agreed with her and kicked the smoking habit.

I hope I have helped convince you that your dentist may directly help you to have better general health by improving your dental health and by early detection of possible medical ailments.

One of the stranger aspects of general health care that I have experienced is the patient who comes in on an emergency visit and tells me that one or two of their upper-back teeth are killing them. The patient often demands or asks to have the tooth extracted because it is so painful. This common complaint should be approached carefully, as the patient's pain might not require dental treatment or tooth extraction. I was trained to perform treatments that are either beneficial or agreed upon by the patient, rather than solely what the patient desires.

I proceed to examine the tooth by observation, testing, and an X-ray to determine whether there is a gum or tooth nerve infection. I also ask the patient what makes it hurt more, hot or cold foods or liquids? If hot drinks or hot foods make the tooth hurt, it usually means there is a tooth nerve infection. Cold sensitivity tells me the nerve is alive. Sometimes, by the time the patient arrives, the pain is gone. Or it comes back when the patient lies down. This symptom tells me it is sinus related. More often than not, this is a classic example of referred pain to the upper-back teeth from a sinus infection. How can this happen?

Anatomically, the origins of the upper-back teeth roots and nerves that travel to the teeth are in the floor of the maxillary sinuses (bony air spaces). When the mucous membrane of the soft tissue lining of the sinus is inflamed or irritated by infection, it can cause referred pain in one or two upper bicuspid or molar teeth, even though those teeth are not diseased. These kinds of complaints happen during the winter season when folks get head colds related to the sinuses. I would see these complaints every year or two.

Of course, upon hearing that this painful tooth is not diseased, the patient is grateful and relieved that it is something else that can be solved by going to a medical specialist and getting a prescription for an antibiotic drug.

This type of scenario goes the other way, too, from

physician to dentist. For example, this can occur when a patient goes to the ear doctor for pain in the ear. On more than one occasion, an otolaryngologist (ear, nose, and throat doctor) referred a patient to me when he found that there was no ear infection. Again, the problem is elsewhere. This can be referred to as pain to the ear originating from the lower molar tooth.

The human body cannot be compartmentalized for treatment by specific dental or medical specialties alone. The body is made up of many different organs, systems, and structures that are interrelated to one another. Since no one doctor can be expected to know every aspect of health care, we doctors divide up and separate areas according to our training of medicine and dentistry. Since we dentists are trained as mouth doctors, we have to know more about the rest of the human body. Our medical colleagues really need to know more about dentistry, but they don't. It has been said—and I have witnessed—that "the mouth can be a picture of a patient's general health."

I was trained and learned to understand the importance of the largest and most complex fifth cranial nerve, the trigeminal nerve, which innervates the teeth. This same nerve is also connected intimately with the surrounding structures of the eye, nose, ear, muscles of mastication (chewing), and sinuses. I learned how pain can be referred from one structure to the other, which can baffle a diagnosis by the dentist or physician.

Or how the infection of the mouth's hard and soft tissues can circulate bacteria throughout the blood system to cause other serious medical diseases. Believe me, when I say periodontal disease is caused by bacteria, and that these oral bacteria can enter the bloodstream and may attach to the fatty plaque in the coronary arteries of the heart. This attachment can result in formation of a blood clot and increases the risk of a variety of health issues, including cardiovascular diseases such as heart attack and stroke, endocarditis, insulin resistance, diabetes, respiratory tract infections, oral and colorectal cancer, pneumonia, middle ear infection and Alzheimer's disease.

In an examination, dentists can learn a lot about their patients' unhealthy habits. I have seen the early signs of alcoholism in a few of my patient's mouths. The oral mucosal tissues of the mouth change from being soft, moist, and glistening pinkish in color to a dry and leathery feel with a gray whitish-pink appearance. Overuse of chewing and smoking tobacco can also change the oral tissues as well. I was even able to detect where a pipe smoker held his pipe—not so much by the teeth, but by the irritation of the palate or inner cheek that would change color and have little red specks all over the area. We all know the consequences of drinking too much alcohol, of heavy smoking, and of using illegal street drugs. These people are four times more likely to get some form of cancer than the general population. As a dental doctor I have seen these changes and shown them to the patient and encouraged them to change these unhealthy habits that can shorten their life. What you don't put in your mouth can be just as important as what you do put in your mouth.

The worst thing you can put in your mouth is the illegal street drug methamphetamine. Over the years only two or three patients with "meth mouth" have consulted me. The total destruction of a young person's teeth and the inflamed lining of their mouth's oral tissues are an unforgettable sight.

The drug is commonly called meth, crank, speed, glass, crystal, quartz, and fire. It is cheap, easy to make, and gives an elation that lasts for up to twelve hours. It also makes the user crave sugary substances, like soda and candy. Users clench or grind their teeth from pain. This often causes teeth to fracture and/or to have severe wear of the dentition, plus a dry mouth. Users will not brush or floss their teeth for several days due to painful and sensitive teeth and gums. This neglect causes decayed teeth and gingivitis. The acidic content of the drug also damages the teeth. It also causes lesions or burns on the lips, gums, inner cheeks, and/or the hard palate.

Meth's other effects on the body are the following: stroke, due to damage of the blood vessels; liver damage, due to the chemicals involved in making the drug; and an increase in body temperature, which can cause brain damage. Use of this drug can weaken the immune system, and the user is unable to fight off infections. Even with all these effects, the user does not experience dental pain because meth can block out the effects of dental pain. Finally, meth can cause death.

A cousin who came to my dental practice when he was a teenager suffered from this drug usage in his twenties. Many of the restorations I did on his teeth not only failed from dental decay, but he lost several teeth. Fortunately, he straightened out his life and survived this destructive drug habit.

Dear reader, when a person has an addiction to

alcohol or tobacco or illegal drugs, is it a medical issue or a dental health issue? Both professions must address these serious health problems. Dental care, which includes the teeth and soft tissues of your mouth, are important for your general health.

Infected teeth and gums, or infection anywhere in the body, can affect the success of organ transplant surgery and other medical conditions that weaken the immune system, such as cardiac valvular surgery or respiratory complaints. The long-term effects of untreated inflammation arising from gingivitis or periodontitis can have an adverse effect on many areas of our body. Because the mouth and all of the associated structures within are connected to the rest of the body, mainly by the vascular or blood system, it is no wonder that our teeth and gums can affect our general health.

Finally, medical researchers are beginning to acknowledge the findings of dental researchers. Although a great deal of research has been done in the past on diseases of the teeth and dental materials, it was not until the 1950s and 1960s that research of the gums (gingival tissues) was done using the electron microscope. This research examined the various types of bacteria located in the gum cuff around the tooth and the spaces between the teeth. Not only were there specific bacteria associated with periodontal disease found in these spaces, but all types of other organisms that can affect one's general well-being.

Up to recent times, medical researchers would not admit that there are links between certain dental diseases and medical diseases that can be precursors for or related to; the exception where this was accepted is preterm, low birth weight infants whose mothers have periodontal disease. What we need is to have medical researchers join dental researchers and conduct their work together. This will result in research projects that have direct joint input so the results may be more certain, such as on the relationship between periodontal disease and diabetes, in which you cannot have one of those diseases for very long, without the other. There may be other, as-yet-unidentified dental and medical diseases that are linked to one another.

This kind of research project will bring the two professions together for the benefit of the patient. After all, as we discussed earlier, it was easy to divide up the body into definite systems or anatomical structures. This was done to train someone to address the ailment and treat it with specialized expertise. We can better manage to prevent and detect early symptoms of diseases when the two professions come together for laboratory research and follow-up clinical trials.

To summarize, although the two professions of dentistry and medicine began separately in the United States, each having their own schools and own training, these professions are joined by human anatomy which does not recognize the separation of what is dental and what is medical.

Your dental care is important to have good general health. We can separate the two professions, but the diseases of the mouth or one part of the body cannot be separated from other parts of the body. A healthy mouth, with healthy teeth and gums, should last a lifetime and can protect you from other medical diseases. As we will see in a later chapter, there is a direct, undeniable relationship between diabetes and periodontal disease.

Let's finish this chapter with a story of teeth in the animal world to discuss why it's important to prevent tooth loss. Teeth are vitally important to an animal's existence. Human beings, as you know, share many similar organs and anatomical structures with other animals. In fact, we are not the only animals to have more than one set of teeth in a lifetime. As you know, humans grow two sets of teeth. Elephants, the largest land animal in the animal kingdom, grow six sets of teeth! Like the human dentition of childhood, the elephant gets a small set of teeth to begin with. Unlike humans, elephants wear out their teeth chewing so much food that they continue to grow five more sets of teeth, replacing the worn-out ones along the way. Unfortunately, upon losing its last set of teeth, an elephant dies of starvation. We need our natural teeth for our overall health and well-being too. Obviously, the very existence of some animals depends on their teeth to capture and eat their prey. As human beings we too depend on our teeth for the mastication of our food to be able to digest meats and hard vegetables. Imagine trying to swallow your food without chewing it.

Thanks to the dental profession, we humans can get along without our natural teeth, but many animals do not do as well. While the situation is less dire for humans if we lose all our teeth, it's far better to practice good oral hygiene. In the next chapter you will learn the importance of devoting a few minutes daily to the necessary homecare and restriction of sweets in your diet.

2

PREVENTION VS. TREATMENT

Ben Franklin said it best: "An ounce of prevention is worth a pound of cure." If I had asked my patients whether they would have liked to prevent a toothache or a gum problem, rather than get treated for it, they would have chosen prevention. It's more pleasant to come in for a regular checkup appointment to prevent problems than to come in for the treatment of problems. Planning and preparation are needed to prevent problems, but it is well worth the effort.

Dental insurance companies can encourage patients to take better courses of action to prevent disease, but these days, they don't. Many years ago, one insurance company, Delta Dental, gave incentives to the California State Teachers Association patients by increasing the dollar amount of coverage for treatment, provided they had wellness checkup visits twice each year and any recommended treatment completed. This incentive to encourage the teachers to pursue more frequent wellness visits resulted in the need for less treatment. This policy had the added benefit of reducing the cost to the patient and to the insurance company—a win-win situation for both parties. Even though most patients understand that prevention is better than treatment, they do not always follow through. Prevention requires advance planning that some people do not make the time for. What is surprising to me is that about 35 percent of the folks that have dental insurance don't regularly go for checkups. They just wait until they think they have a problem.

The two most common dental problems requiring treatment are cavities and gum disease, such as gingivitis. Most children, teenagers, and young adults have cavities during their early years until they are twenty to twenty-five years old. Then they figure out that they should not consume so many sweet things like candy and sodapop. Later in life, after age thirty-five, the most common problems are tooth loss from advanced gum disease. Proper oral hygiene at home and avoiding a lot of sweets helps prevent problems. With regular dental wellness checkups, these diseases can be prevented or treated early to prevent tooth loss.

I recommend semiannual checkups to most of my patients. To allow for early detection of disease, these checkups include cleaning; an examination, sometimes with X-rays; and screening for oral cancer. This schedule is especially important for patients who are prone to decay or heavy tartar deposits. Early detection could mean the difference between a patient needing a filling instead of a crown. Early detection of gingivitis can prevent a more serious condition called periodontitis, which involves gum recession around the teeth and the loss of bone—and possibly the loss of teeth. For some patients, a more frequent preventive visit schedule is recommended, and even with these added visits, dental costs are lower with preventive care. To help patients stay on schedule with their preventive care, my office staff would call our patients to remind them of their need for a preventive checkup appointment.

In 1913 the dental profession started an auxiliary dental hygienist training program to do dental hygiene care. Teeth cleaning of calculus or tartar on an annual or semiannual basis is done to prevent gum disease. It was believed that calculus or tartar was the irritant that caused gum diseases. However, in the 1960s, the contrast phase and electron microscopes revealed that the tartar or calculus that accumulates on our teeth is not what causes irritation that leads to gingivitis. What causes gum disease is bacterial plaque (biofilm) that sticks to calculus. Not the tartar alone.

Unfortunately, during a wellness visit, professionally trained dental hygienists are not given enough time to teach patients proper and necessary flossing, in addition to brushing. They only have time to clean your teeth and help find cavities and gum problems for the dentist to treat. All dentists and hygienists agree and know that gingivitis, the first stage of periodontitis, can be remedied by proper flossing, in addition to brushing daily. Brushing alone does not remove the bacterial plaque (biofilm) that can cause dental decay, plus gum and bone diseases. The irritant that causes these problems is found between the teeth and in the crevice between the tooth and gum cuff—where the toothbrush cannot reach. Interdental (between the teeth) areas must be cleaned with proper flossing or other interdental devices, which require professional instruction as well.

Periodic bitewing X-ray examinations can detect decay of an existing filling. Recurrent decay is when a new cavity is formed in the area that was treated. Dental decay may recur because no filling, crown, or veneer can be completely seal or bond to the tooth in an airtight manner. Unless you change or improve your dietary habits and oral hygiene habits to create a neutral saliva and remove the biofilm sticking to your teeth daily, you may continue to have cavities and/or the silent dental disease of gingivitis, or worse, periodontitis. These diseases of the teeth and gums will respond positively to better oral hygiene practices at home. However, early detection is the key to maintaining a lifelong healthy dentition (teeth).

What I am saying here is that it is important for patients to learn that almost all dental restorative treatments of the teeth and gums are still subject to the continuation of the disease processes. The dental treatment you receive gives you a second chance to prevent the recurrence of disease, which you can do with improved oral hygiene and the reduction of sweets in your diet. Let me summarize by what I used to tell my patients when redoing some dental work. "There isn't anything I can do, that you, as my patient, cannot undo." Fillings or restorations may need to be replaced, not because of wearing out, but more often because of recurrent decay.

As an undergraduate, before I had the chance to learn about tooth and gum diseases in dental school, I studied anthropology. I have always wondered how much of what we know about prehistoric humans comes from the buried archaeological remains of early Homo sapiens jawbones and teeth. Anthropologists have found teeth that have remained intact for over nine hundred thousand years. And yet, in our time, some people cannot retain and keep their teeth from being diseased or extracted in less than seventy-five years of life. And it's even more surprising when you consider that nowadays in the US, we have plenty of access to dental care: there are about two hundred thousand practicing American dentists, many of whom are ready and waiting to take care of people with dental problems.

Dental practitioners often complete their treatment by providing instructions or demonstrations on how to maintain the treatment received. I know that doing the treatment is easier than trying to change your home care or eating habits. I also know that doing the treatment is easier than training you to floss your teeth along with brushing. However, very few insurance companies will allow payment for oral hygiene instructions (OHI) more than once a year. Receiving an annual or biannual demonstration of flossing techniques from your dentist or hygienist is insufficient. Teaching a patient how to floss properly requires four to eight appointments over a month's time.

As a child, I had bad eating habits, consuming candy, ice cream and sodapop almost daily. My mother used to make sweet Armenian pastries, which we had in the pantry all year round. Besides, there was a candy store on my block that I had to pass twice a day on my way to grammar school. As a result, even though I had dental care from the age of seven or eight, I had a lot of fillings. Never did a day pass when I didn't have candy, sodapop, or pastries. Every time I went to the dentist, I had to have more fillings. The combination of my poor dental condition and my sister's job choice was how I decided to become a dentist. Here is my story:

When my older sister became a dental assistant, the first dentist she worked for was a nice man in North Beach, a neighborhood in San Francisco. So, my father told us to go to him—even though it was across town. Looking back on my treatment now, it's clear to me that he was a "drill, fill, and bill dentist." At every checkup appointment, I had more decayed (redecayed) teeth. He never gave me any advice about how to take better care of my teeth. Fortunately, my sister left his practice after a couple of years and started working for Dr. T. Galt Atwood at 450 Sutter Street, which was around the block from Union Square and closer to home. By the age of fifteen years old, most of my back teeth and some of my front ones had restorations (fillings).

On my first appointment with Dr. Atwood, he said that he had to replace an existing filling because the tooth had decayed. After removing the decay and old filling, he told me there was a problem: there was not very much of the tooth left to hold the new larger filling. I told him that I had bad teeth. He said, "No, you don't have bad teeth; you are just putting bad things in your mouth. You are eating too many sweet things like candy, gum, ice creme, soda pop, cookies, and cakes." All of what he said was true! He continued, "If you stop eating a lot of these sweet snack foods, you can stop having these cavities."

Well, right then and there, I swore off eating these sweet things that were causing me dental problems. When I went back for a six-month checkup with bitewing X-rays, I did not have any new cavities. I was proud of myself and told my dentist that my visits to him were bad for his business. He stated that this was incorrect because he had numerous other tasks for his other patients. He was pleased that I had no recurrent decay and that his main job was to help people to have healthier teeth and gums. Hearing that response made me want to become a dentist like him.

Dr. Atwood became my role model and my mentor. This personal relationship that developed between patient and doctor is necessary for behavior change of the patient's dietary and oral hygiene habits. In my experience, very few children and adults can have the discipline to change bad eating habits for good ones in a brief time. It usually takes a longer-term relationship with your dentist to make a change in your diet or oral hygiene habits.

Of all the possible diseases we face throughout our lifetime, cavities and gum problems are the most common and can remain a problem for the rest of our life. Dental caries (decay) of children's teeth is the most prevalent chronic childhood disease known. It affects 99 percent of children worldwide, according to the Global Burden of Disease 2021. Therefore, early and frequent dental visits are necessary to detect and prevent a painful experience or the early loss of a child's tooth. So-called "baby teeth" are the primary teeth, some of which must remain in the child's mouth until they are thirteen years old. This allows the secondary adult dentition to align in the proper places. A diseased child's tooth can transfer disease to adult teeth. From the ages of six to fourteen a child has a mixed dentition of primary and secondary teeth. This is the reason a child's first set of teeth are just as important as the secondary dentition that must last for the rest of one's life.

Disease transfer happens because acidic saliva, bacterial plaque, and sugary foods or drinks in the diet remain unchanged. Many parents do not realize that children's teeth enamel is half as thick as adult teeth, providing less protection against decay reaching the dentin and nerve.

Another fact that many parents do not realize is that the more sweets a child consumes the more the child wants. A heavily sugary diet is addictive. It is common knowledge that sweets are the main cause of decay of the teeth at all ages. (Chocolate lovers beware.) Many packaged snacks are laden with sugar. The biggest offender that I know so well is the breakfast cereals. Only one or two of these cereals have acceptable amounts of sugar or no sugar at all.

For snacks, I recommend for my patients to choose a vegetable, some fruit, or nuts, as these whole foods have complex sugars and carbohydrates that do not break down easily in the mouth. Instead, they break down in the stomach (gut). Soda drinkers have a choice of diet sodas, which help them avoid the typical content of about eleven teaspoons of sugar in a twelve-ounce can (not to mention the unwanted calories). Is it any wonder that the richest country in the world has the highest rate of diabetes? One of my nutritional science course professors in dental school would say that what you don't put in your mouth may be more important than what you do.

For example, one of my patients referred a young woman to my care. She was a flight attendant who worked for a foreign airline. She lived in Austria but was domiciled in San Francisco. Her complaint was that she had extreme sensitivity to her teeth from cold foods and beverages. Sometimes all her teeth just ached. I did a complete examination of full-mouth X-rays and a visual clinical examination of her mouth, teeth, and gums; no decay was present. I could only detect extreme sensitivity to her teeth with cold water and cold air. So, I asked her to go back to my reception room and sit down and record all the food and drinks she had consumed that day and the previous day, listing them under breakfast, lunch, and dinner. My staff gave her a clipboard, writing paper, and a pen.

When she was through and I read what she had written, I was surprised that she was drinking a lot of tea. She was drinking eight or more cups each day using honey to sweeten the tea. So, I asked her how much honey she put into each cup. She told me that she only put two teaspoons of honey in each cup. This totaled an average of sixteen teaspoons of honey daily. I asked her which size bottle of honey she would purchase. She said that she was buying a gallon can of honey since it was so much more reasonably priced. She told me that honey was expensive in her home country and not easily available in that quantity. At this point, I had to try and hide my astonishment at what she was doing. I told her that the honey was the cause of her teeth sensitivity. She had to immediately reduce the amount of honey that she was consuming to solve her problem. Otherwise, she would cause decay of the roots and crowns of her teeth. She protested, at first, telling me that the honey was organic. I informed her that honey is a supersaturated solution of refined sucrose, which could cause significant harm to her teeth beyond just pain.

I advised her to gradually reduce her tea consumption and use less honey until she could stop entirely. I suggested nonsugar sweeteners as substitutes and asked for weekly progress reports. She was recommended to rinse her mouth with warm water immediately after each honey-sweetened cup of tea. I also recommended desensitizing toothpaste, which was available at the time, telling her that the reversal of sensitivity takes time. It took about six or seven weeks before she weaned herself off honey and stopped the sensitivity of her teeth.

Extensive research conducted over many years has significantly advanced our understanding of the chemical processes involved in dental caries (decay). Our saliva is important in protecting our teeth by maintaining a neutral pH (acidity). We know that decay advances best in an acid environment of the mouth. When we eat something, the remains of the food on our teeth change the saliva to become acidic. To lessen this acid saliva, if you can't brush immediately after a meal or snack, I would tell my patients that they can rinse their mouth with water to help the saliva return to a neutral acidity. Of course, snacking between meals can promote decay, particularly if the food contains flour or sugar.

Oral hygiene with an oral irrigator can give you a false sense of cleaning the in-between of your teeth because it removes particles of food. But this device cannot remove the sticky bacterial plaque (biofilm) that is the causative factor of cavities and gum diseases. Due to misleading advertising and insufficient research, this device has been recommended by some dentists for home care.

Fortunately, today there are several preventive procedures by your dentist that can be done to avoid or prevent having a decayed tooth besides avoiding sweets. For children's teeth, a procedure called sealants can be applied to the chewing surface of a molar or of bicuspid back teeth: a possible pit in a tooth's enamel can be sealed to avoid decay. This type of treatment can be done without local anesthesia, in other words, no injection or shot of medication. Children must be at least six years old to allow their cooperation because the tooth chewing surfaces must be cleaned and dried before application. The child's mouth must be kept open for about five minutes. Usually, a child's first molar teeth emerge between six to seven years of age. These adult molar teeth are the keystones of the upper and lower dental arches. They guide all the other back adult teeth to align properly in the dental arches.

Most children I have treated benefited from the preventive procedures that insurance companies do not cover. For instance, the application of a strong fluoride gel to teeth that exhibit some decalcification of the enamel can recalcify the enamel. It may also be used if the child or teenager has an elevated risk or propensity for decay. I would prescribe medication to my patients for a daily rinse of fluoride gel at home. This potent gel could reverse the decalcification of the enamel, which is the beginning stage of developing a cavity.

Another preventive procedure that I have learned since graduation is the use of caries risk assessment (CRA). This evaluation can prevent dental caries before they occur. I was not trained to evaluate the degree of decay and the likelihood of the need for future treatment. Now my dental students, just like oncologists who evaluate different stages of a cancerous tumor, can evaluate the degree of decay in a tooth. In this way, dentists can determine the various stages of penetration of the decay into the enamel, or even dentin, of the tooth. In early detection of incipient decay, the dentist can wait and see if the patient is willing to improve their oral hygiene practices and dietary habits to avoid the progression of the decay. Dental caries detection by using CRA can help decide which teeth to watch and which teeth to treat.

Years ago, I was trained to treat all signs of decay. We used to think decay couldn't be stopped once it began. The present research now proves that beginning decay of the teeth can be stopped—not only in the enamel, but also in the inner layer of dentin of the tooth.

I have been able to follow one of my adult daughter's dental conditions. During her teenage years she began eating more sugary foods and developed incipient decay. This decay penetrated the enamel into the dentin. I showed her these areas of three of her bicuspid teeth on the bitewing X-rays. I told her that if she ate fewer sweets and did more regular and thorough flossing, she could avoid having some fillings.

Today, she sometimes must remind her new dentist that the decay areas on the new X-rays have not changed. The decay has been stopped and no treatment is required.

For the last twenty-five years, a chemical called silver diamine fluoride (SDF) has been available.

Dental schools teach using SDF to halt tooth decay. A small amount of SDF medicament is placed on the decayed area after removal of the decay. The final restoration is placed. Miraculously, the decay process is stopped by a healing process called secondary dentin which will be formed to protect the dental pulp (nerve). Discovery and usage of SDF has created another revolutionary advancement for the prevention and control of dental decay.

But again, this is not to say that a patient cannot still cause decay to recur from lack of proper oral hygiene and/or frequency of snacking with candy, sugary foods, and sugary drinks. Brushing twice a day, after breakfast and dinner, plus flossing after dinner is still the best way to prevent tooth and gum diseases.

The efficacy of flossing was established by the research of Dr. Harald Loe. He was a Norwegian dental educator and periodontal researcher. He conducted research demonstrating that gingivitis, a precursor to periodontitis, can develop from not brushing or flossing for two weeks. Then the disease process is reversed and remedied by resuming brushing and flossing. His research was titled "Experimental Gingivitis in Man." This research finding was pivotal. Why do I say this? Periodontal. Res 1: 1-13,1966

Because up to this time, the dental profession believed that tartar (calculus) on the teeth was the cause of gum inflammation. But instead, it is the biofilm stuck to the tartar that is the cause of gingivitis. You must know how to floss properly to get rid of this gum irritation, but most people do not floss properly because they were never trained or taught by an especially trained dental professional.

I remember many years ago the efficacy of flossing was challenged. This resulted in an extended controversy. Countless studies were repeated to show that brushing alone did not remove the biofilm in the in-between spaces. Finally, the consensus of these studies proved that dental flossing could prevent gingivitis and control periodontitis to some degree.

Unfortunately, all toothpastes, mouthwashes, and oral irrigators that are advertised on TV by major dental product manufacturers, or recommended by some dentists, do not remove the sticky biofilm. The biofilm is between the tooth and in the cuff of gum surrounding each tooth. What bothers me is that some of these companies have received the certification of the ADA. These companies are not warned to stop the false advertising by the ADA. Why the ADA does not threaten these companies with certification withdrawal is a wonder to me.

I have observed that many children and young adults can have healthy gums, free from bleeding, without the use of daily flossing. The immune system or growth hormones of younger people can resist the irritation of the bacterial colonies that produce chemical poisons. However, after about the late teens or early twenties, gum health changes and inflammation can be detected by bleeding gums. First, the bleeding from gum inflammation starts between the back teeth. Later, it progresses to the front teeth. All adults who do not use floss daily have some bleeding areas between their back teeth and sometimes even their front teeth. During my four decades of dental practice, I have only seen three or four patients who do not floss and have no bleeding gums.

Many of my older patients are often concerned about the recession of their gums. Both adults and seniors can develop normal recession of healthy gum tissues. If the recession is simply due to aging, this is normal. However, recession can also be due to long-standing gum disease. Receding gum tissues allow more interdental space between the teeth, which allows food impaction. I have helped my patients choose the proper type of floss or other cleaning devices, such as tiny interdental brushes or Stim-U-Dents. Many types of floss can expand and clean the larger spaces between the teeth.

I always tell my dental students when they are asking about their patients' oral hygiene habits, don't ask your patients if they floss their teeth. Just give them the floss and ask them to show you what they are doing with it. Most patients will tell the dentist that they use dental floss, but they might only use it when they have just eaten corn on the cob or some stringy meat that got stuck between their teeth. Not daily. Or they just floss their front teeth because the back ones are too hard to get to. Once you see what a patient is doing with the floss, then you realize that most patients do not floss correctly or thoroughly. Proper flossing does not come naturally. A patient must be taught how to use dental floss properly. I like to state the fact that the word "doctor" was derived from the word for teacher. Your dentist or staff members, such as, dental assistant or therapist, should teach you how to floss properly.

I trained a dental therapist in my office who conducted a one-on-one program for five consecutive days, allowing twenty-five-to-thirty-minute appointments. Then the patient would return the following week, once or twice, to see if the patient was still improving their technique. Later, after one month, they would return to show the therapist what they learned. In my estimation, it takes about four to eight visits to train someone how to use floss properly. If insurance companies covered oral hygiene instructions (OHI), teaching oral hygiene in dental offices would increase.

I have learned from my patients that folks do not usually lose teeth all at once, but instead, one at a time. Some patients say they cannot afford root canal treatment. Yet the cost of prevention is so much less. For instance, the annual cost of two visits per year might range, depending on the location, from two hundred to three hundred dollars. Most one-visit fillings would cost more. A crown would cost about three or four times more than the cost of a filling or restoration. Preventive services, whether for your car maintenance or for your dental health, are always less costly than the repair or treatment.

So how does loss of a tooth happen?

An old dental adage goes like this: For lack of brushing and flossing, the patient develops a cavity. For lack of a filling, the decay spreads to other parts of the tooth and requires a crown. For lack of a crown, the decay progresses to infect the nerve. For lack of root canal therapy, the tooth is painful and/or infected and must be extracted.

The loss of teeth from gum problems usually occurs after the age of thirty-five. If a patient of mine has gum pocket depths, within the cuff of gum around the tooth, of 4 mm or more, plus more than three or four bleeding sites of the gums, with no loss of bone or looseness of the teeth, this is diagnosed as gingivitis. Gingivitis can be reversed. I would promise the patient a stoppage of the bleeding in five to ten days. The pocket depths would often be reduced after about four to six weeks. All these results could be attained by thoroughly flossing properly. Of course, I recommend rinsing and brushing first before flossing. I also recommend the use of disclosing tablets that show where the bacterial plaque may remain after brushing without using toothpaste. Disclosing tablets stain the bacterial plaque to a reddish-blue color that is otherwise not visible. The colored saliva solution, which results from the chewed tablet and squishing around in the mouth for a minute, reveals the missed plaque areas. Disclosing tablets can be purchased at most drug stores or ask your dentist for some.

Like any other hand skill, flossing takes practice. Once you know how to do it properly, it takes about four minutes or less. You often hear the recommendation from your dentist or the American Dental Association about the need to brush for two minutes, twice daily. Why is flossing not mentioned or the importance of it in addition to brushing? Especially since the biofilm between our teeth has more bacteria and is more virulent than that on the outer aspects of our teeth. The fact is that flossing is more important in controlling or preventing gum disease than brushing. Still, the ADA continues to give inadequate advice about caring for your teeth and gums.

The January-February 11, 2024, issue of Consumer Reports magazine had a pretty good eight-page article on keeping teeth and gums healthy. However, I do not agree with the comment that brushing is more beneficial than flossing—the article stated that the scientific evidence for flossing is not as strong as brushing. I vehemently disagree. To settle this question, I am curious what your dentist would say?

The best person to ask for an opinion of whether you are in control of bacterial plaque (biofilm) on your teeth is your hygienist or dentist. Assess your home care routine at every preventive visit.

Without a doubt, prevention trumps treatment every time. Think about all the things we do to prevent injury from an automobile accident, such as the mandatory use of safety belts. In California, we have laws that require us to replace our car tires when the tread thickness reaches 2 / 32 of an inch, so there is enough rubber tread to stop in time to prevent an accident. Or the fact that you buy health insurance to prevent the high cost of hospitalization in case you need an operation or serious illness. Would a homeowner not afford to buy fire insurance to prevent loss of his home? In fact, if you have a mortgage on your home, it is mandatory to have a homeowner's policy that includes fire insurance. Insurance can make good business sense.

Preventive dental care means having regular wellness visits or checkups to detect dental problems before something hurts in your mouth. Or before you feel some pain when you bite on something hard. Or before one or all your teeth become sensitive. Or before you notice blood on your toothbrush or floss. Because by the time you notice something hurts, often it is too late to prevent some treatment.

Or perhaps it is gum treatment, such as deep periodontal scaling or periodontal surgery by your dentist or periodontist. Yet several years later, your gum problem returns with deeper-than-normal pockets around the teeth.

What happens is this. The biofilm begins to organize colonies of bacteria on the tooth's surface within twenty-four to forty-eight hours; it must be disorganized daily by flossing. This daily effort prevents the detrimental effects of the chemical toxins that biofilm can produce. It is these chemical poisons that irritate the thin tissues until rupture of the skin barrier and bleeding occurs. Thereby, inflammatory bacteria of the gum tissues can travel throughout the rest of the body by the circulatory blood system to all your vital organs.

Another good reason for regular checkups is that other than a dentist, very few physicians are trained to examine and recognize oral cancer. Oral cancer has a high morbidity rate. This is because it is often undetected due to infrequent dental visits. Once it has progressed in an area close to the vital structures of the neck and brain, the consequences can result in extensive disfiguring surgery or worse, the loss of life. Thus, cancer screening examinations can add a life-saving value to a routine dental visit.

Interestingly, there are studies that prove the historic processing of sugarcane and sugar beets, making sugar more accessible and affordable, have been responsible for the increase of dental caries throughout the world. Moreover, sugar was a preservative for foods that was used to preserve storage foods on long ocean voyages.. The same is true for the processing and refinement of wheat to make white flour for cakes and bread. In fact, removing the bran from the wheat kernel robbed this grain of most of its nutritional value. So much so, that the Department of Agriculture, in the early 1900s, had to pass a regulation that most flour had to have certain vitamins added so the consumer avoided malnutrition. The abundance of both sugar and flour, being highly processed foods, has been the cause of increased dental caries worldwide.

To sum up, the success of dental treatment depends on what you eat and how well you remove food and bacteria from your teeth afterwards.

Dental surgery is unique. Compared to medical surgery, the success of dental treatment depends on home care of the teeth and gums by the patient—for the rest of their life. Consider the occurrence of appendicitis, an inflammation of the diseased appendix, which must be removed. What does the medical surgeon ask that you do postoperatively? Nothing, besides taking it easy for a few days or weeks. After this operation, a friend of mine was back playing tennis the following week.

Yes, there are some medical surgeries that require the patient to do things differently for a while. If, for instance, you have rotator cuff repair or hip surgery, you must follow up with several weeks of physical therapy for the best result. But none of these surgeries require you to perform hygiene once or twice a day, in an area of your body that is very difficult to see and clean properly, like the teeth inside of your mouth.

But then again, it's not surprising that many dental patients aren't taught the importance of prevention to prevent the need for re-treatment. Especially when dental students themselves aren't being educated properly on the importance either. This issue and more will be discussed later in chapter 4 on dental school education.

The next chapter is about the public health policy of community water fluoridation. I believe this public health measure has prevented more cavities among children than all the two hundred thousand dentists in the country can do in their offices.

3

FLUORIDATION: METHODS AND BENEFITS

Community water fluoridation (CWF) is the addition of a micronutrient, fluoride, to a water-supply system to provide a health benefit for the population: the strengthening of the enamel of the teeth, which in turn, helps teeth to resist cavities. This first began in the United States in the late 1940s and early 1950s. Fluoridation was declared to be one of the ten most important public health measures of the twentieth century. At the time, it was known that the addition of this trace element could reduce cavities by 40 to 60 percent in children and young people between the ages of one-to-twenty-five years. It also has a limited beneficial effect on reducing cavities for adult teeth.

During the late 1940s, the American population numbered about 200 million people. At best, CWF would only reach about half of the American population because only about half the population was living in large cities and towns with water-supply systems. CWF is an expensive service, so implementation depends on a community size of at least thirty-five thousand people to keep the cost at an acceptable amount per person. Of the 100 million people after receiving CWF, only about 25 percent (25 million) were children and young adults who would benefit from CWF.

My own three children, here in San Francisco, had the benefits of CWF in the late 1960s. As a result, my two daughters have fewer than six cavities between them, and my son has never had a cavity. Although I did not treat a lot of children in my dental practice, I saw significant improvement to the children I treated in dental school some eight years earlier. The children in CWF areas can achieve healthy teeth along with daily oral hygiene and reduction of sweets. With a more resistant tooth enamel, the incidence of cavities in children is reduced by half and the tooth decay process is slowed. This allows children to improve their oral hygiene and for parents to have lower dental treatment costs.

Public implementation of CWF did not happen overnight. From the discovery to the implementation of CWF took forty-five years of research that depended on many people. The method of evaluating the water where a large concentration of fluoride existed had to be advanced. The technology of water-measurement instruments had to be developed. It is one thing to measure how many parts per million of an element are present in the water. It is another thing to add just one part per million parts of that element to a water-supply system.

How was this miraculous element, fluoride, discovered? In 1901, a young dentist named Dr. Frederick S. McKay, of Colorado Springs, Colorado, saw that some of his younger patients had an unusual permanent brown stain on their teeth. Many of the residents called it "Colorado brown stain." However, McKay also observed that the teeth affected by this condition seemed to have fewer cavities—or none. He was inquisitive enough to figure out that it was something they were drinking or eating. He then reported his findings by informing other dentists outside of the area by word of mouth or through articles in dental journals. Other dentists outside of his area began reporting the same phenomenon. Dr. McKay spent the rest of his life researching and working with the dental profession to bring CWF to the public.

The so-called brown strain was a result of a very heavy concentration of fluoride in the water. Most elements, be they fluoride, copper, or magnesium, have a color. Please note, though, that when the amount of these elements—fluoride, in particular—is very small, reduced to one milligram or less, it does not cause discoloration in children's teeth.

How does CFW work? The crystalline structure of enamel prefers to be attached to the fluoride ion (F), when present, rather than to the hydroxyl ion (OH) that is normally in the apatite crystalline structure of enamel. So, the fluoride ion replaces the hydroxyl ion. When the fluoride ion is present in the water supply, it only requires 0.7 to- 1.0 milligrams of fluoride per million parts of water for the tooth enamel becomes more resistant to decay. This phenomenon took years of research to evaluate and implement.

Finally, by 1945, the American Dental Association formed a team of dental researchers who started taking samples of the water and testing the water to determine which minerals were present. They found out that in some places the water contained nine to twelve parts of fluoride per million parts of water. This was a very large and unusual amount, as fluoride is usually a trace of mineral in water, much less than one part per million. Dental researchers proved that all that was needed in the drinking water was about one part per million or less to harden the tooth enamel, so it resists decay. But most available water does not have enough fluoride to harden the tooth enamel. So, the least amount of fluoride determined to be adequate was 0.7 milligrams of fluoride per 1 million parts of water.

However, CWF has its limits. The first sign of developing teeth begins in utero in newborn infants. (Interestingly, the tooth structure beginning (germ) is evident and in the embryo from the fourth or fifth month of pregnancy.) Ideally, a pregnant mother needs to have fluoride in her diet to achieve the maximum benefit of fluoridation. Thereafter, children may benefit from the presence of fluoride in their diet up to the age of twenty-five. Adults with fully formed teeth also benefit from the presence of fluoride in their diet, but to a lesser degree.

Unfortunately, since the inception of CWF seventy-nine years ago, with the increase in our population, only about 63 percent of the population has been able to have the advantages of fewer dental caries through the benefits of CWF. This is because CWF is only available in larger populated communities. Children and young adults living in small or rural communities or using well water cannot benefit from this great public health measure. Therefore, we have reached the maximum penetration or saturation of CWF.

Children and young people are not the only people to benefit from CFW. Senior citizens also receive the benefit of water fluoridation when they have decreased saliva and an inability to wash away food from their teeth. Their teeth will form senile caries or hyper fluoridated areas which do not decay. So, seniors living in major cities and larger communities receive the public health benefit of CWF too. I have estimated that, considering our population of about 340 million people, over 85 million children and young adults suffer from a public health disparity. This limited availability of CWF has not only created a huge dental health disparity between city families and agricultural and rural families, but these families from agricultural and rural areas are often folks who can least afford the cost of dental treatment for their children.

Even though the data of the Centers for Disease Control and Prevention (CDC) shows that CWF use has not increased in the past decade, the ADA, the US Public Health Services, and the Food and Drug Administration (FDA) have doggedly held on to only one kind of fluoridation. Why does this matter? Because there is another option that is available for reaching more of our children and young adults with another kind of fluoridation. This option will be discussed next.

Community Resistance and Other Challenges to Fluoridated Water

There has been controversy and opposition to CWF and its public health benefit from the beginning. In fact, there are still several organizations today that believe that fluoridated water can cause health problems. Communities all over the country have had debates on the issue of whether to fluoridate the community water supply, as they said that it only helped children and young people. Yet it is the older folks who are the taxpayers of any increase in costs from this public health benefit. What emerged from these debates was a group of people called "antifluoridationists." They went around the country wherever community meetings were considering the implementation of CWF and vehemently spoke against it. They would try to scare away people with false research and statistics by saying that adding fluoride to the water causes mental deficiencies in children's brains.

When I was a dental student in the early 1960s, the local dentists were advised not to attend these community meetings. The ADA had a cadre of public health dental scientists and spokespeople who were assigned to attend these meetings and argue against the antifluoridationists. The ADA didn't want the local dentists to participate as they might be viewed as having a special interest or benefit, rather than being there to benefit the public. That was the thinking at the time because there were a handful of dentists who were opposed to CWF. I believe they may have felt that a reduction in cavities would affect their bottom line. The only dentists I know who noticed less business in CWF areas were the pediatric dentists who treated children and teenagers. After a while, they began doing more interceptive orthodontics and stayed busy. I don't know of any dentist who had significant loss of income from fewer cavities to fill.

In order to implement CWF, the ADA had to lobby and persuade these municipalities to place CWF on the ballot to get permission from the electorate to alter the public water supply by adding this micronutrient to it . This started the antifluoridationist wars. This group of people felt that putting a microchemical in the water supply was the same as medicating the water supply. Of course, they did not recognize that all community water sources are chlorinated for the prevention of some very serious diseases. Besides, they argued, why should we be washing our cars and watering our lawns with fluoridated water? This argument made sense to some of the people then.

The ADA was so maligned and maliciously and falsely accused of harming children's health with CWF that they decided to let other agencies take over. The promotion and record keeping of those communities that implemented CWF, as well as those that were debating the issue, was passed on to the CDC and the US Public Health Service (USPHS). Besides accusing the ADA of medicating the water, the antifluoridationists produced bogus research to try and justify their claim that harm would come to the children from CWF.

For instance, there is a very rare kidney disease that affects less than one-tenth of one percent of the American population—people who are allergic to fluoride and can become ill from small amounts of fluoride. The physicians of these folks know to warn their patients not to drink fluoridated water. The antifluoridationists used this condition and maintained that fluoride affects most children adversely, even though they do not have this kidney illness.

It is the CDC and the USPHS that are charged with monitoring the percentage of people receiving CWF. These two agencies maintain a periodic recordkeeping of the questionable increase in CWF. I believe that the dental profession can and should do better than just turn over the recordkeeping of CWF to these agencies. The ADA should not give a deaf ear to cities that have decided against providing CWF for assorted reasons. Let me share some examples of where that is happening in the US.

The California Dental Foundation, of the CDA, wanted to increase CWF throughout the state. It targeted Santa Clara County, which includes Silicon Valley and the City of San Jose. The program started in 2012, and the goal was to implement fluoridation for two-thirds of the county by 2017. A facility costing $8 million dollars was estimated to be needed to start the program to implement CWF in the growing San Jose area near Silicon Valley. As time went on, the costs increased to $16 million dollars. Here is a growing four-million-person population that had plans for more money to put fluoride into the water supply systems. The state was also going to contribute money along the way. As time to accumulate the funds went on, the costs continued to increase. As of 2024, the project is still on the planning table and not in operation. The costs of starting a new facility to implement community water fluoridation, not to mention the maintenance cost of the program, are no longer affordable.

There has been some growing resistance to continuing CWF in some communities due to it increasing maintenance costs. For example, the region of Tampa-St. Petersburg, Florida, and the city of Dallas, Texas, went back and forth on this issue until they established the funds to continue to fluoridate the water. Finally, the voters, who are mainly senior citizens, gave in to the younger families who wanted their children to have the benefits of fewer cavities.

What is more alarming is the discontinuation of CWF. Portland, Oregon comes to mind. The community there voted several times to reestablish CWF but was defeated by a vote of 60 percent to 40 percent. The people there want a natural supply of water and in their minds, it should not be medicated.

Davis, California, a college town of sixty-five thousand that is noted for its highly educated and liberal residents, recently stands out. This town is home to the University of California, at Davis . The city had never fluoridated water before; they had numerous well-water sources. Now with an expensive project of bringing water from the Sacramento River, the question of adding fluoride was to be decided by a committee of the city council. The council included Dr. Howard Pollick, who is a professor of dental public health from UC, San Francisco's dental school. Dr. Pollick reported that the committee recommended fluoridation to the city council. In spite of this recommendation, the city council voted four to one to not add fluoride to the water. Dr. Pollick was disappointed in this result. He has seen more cities, including Santa Cruz, Redding, and Modesto, reject fluoridation. And other cities, such as Oroville, have discontinued fluoridation after years of adding fluoride to the water.

The debate over whether to fluoridate the drinking water in Honolulu, Hawaii, has raged for decades. In 2004, the city and county voters supported a fluoridation ban by a vote of five to one. They believe their water, air, and soil are pure and should not be altered. Now the only places in Honolulu that can have water fluoridation are on military bases.

Introducing Salt Fluoridation

There is another kind of fluoridation that uses table salt. It is called salt fluoridation. I first learned about this other form of fluoridation when I read a book entitled Promoting Oral Health: The Use of Salt Fluoridation to Prevent Dental Caries, by Saskia Estupiñán-Day in 2005. It is the only book I have found on the subject of salt fluoridation in the United States. Moreover, many American-trained public dentists I have met have no knowledge of salt fluoridation. The ones whom I have met who do know about it look down their noses at its usage. Furthermore, they like to say the CWF is the gold standard.

Switzerland has used salt fluoridation for over 75 years. In fact, salt fluoridation is used in several European countries, such as Germany, Austria, France, Poland, Belarus, Greece, and Hungary. It is also used in more than twenty Central and South American countries. As many countries use salt fluoridation (SF) as use CWF. Many countries produce table salt that is both iodized and fluoridated since these elements are compatible. In some of the countries that produce fluoridated salt, it is the only kind of salt available. In other countries there is a choice of other types of salt.

Why can't Americans buy table salt that is iodized and fluoridated to improve their dental health? Because the American Dental Association (ADA), on their website, purports that CWF is the most effective way to curtail dental caries. Moreover, the ADA says that CWF is the most cost-effective way to control cavities. Neither of these statements is true. Salt fluoridation (SF) is the most cost-effective way to introduce fluoride into the diet. Another reason that the purchase of fluoridated table salt is not available is that the FDA will not allow it to be produced in the United States.

In her book, Estupinan-Day claims that SF is eighty to one hundred times cheaper than CWF. This contrasts with the ADA's statement about the cost-effectiveness of CWF. In addition, the ADA continues to ignore the fact that about 35 percent of the children and adults in this country will never be able to have CWF due to the lack of water-supply systems capable of delivering water fluoridation.

One reason for opposing the sale and availability of iodized and fluoridated table salt is the concern about causing fluorosis in younger children. Fluorosis is the cosmetic change in the tooth enamel with white spots or tea stains. This likelihood is remote, at best. Because it requires a family living in a non-CWF area to move to a CWF area and bring along their box of fluoridated table salt. Thus, their child would get much more than the recommended amount of fluoride. With fluoride in both the water and in the salt, the combined amount may cause fluorosis on some of the front teeth of children under six years of age.

Salt fluoridation will be unsuitable for use in areas with community water fluoridation. Even today, all toothpaste brands containing fluoride have labels warning that children under six years old must have parental supervision on its usage. Another level of oversight may include the fact that most supermarket supply buyers would not want to buy a product that is not to be used in their area. The use of a warning label should prevent the chance of exposure to more than one source of fluoride.

Once fluoridated salt is available in the US, it will be just as efficacious as community water fluoridation. What I am saying is that the US's rural population can use fluoridated salt instead of CWF and receive the same benefits for their children, with no public investment. Both types of fluoridation would reach the entire population. However, aside from the large initial costs of CWF, as described in California, there is a continuing annual maintenance cost. Salt fluoridation differs, and could be available on every grocery store shelf, except in areas of CWF, if the FDA made it available.

Without a doubt, the children and adults of Hawaii would benefit from the purchase and use of fluoridated salt. And there would be no conflict with CWF to possibly cause fluorosis. With this in mind, several years ago, I met the regent from the American College of Dentists (ACD) from Honolulu, through a mutual friend at our West Coast-area component meeting. He was our guest lecturer at my Northern California component of the ACD in San Francisco. I met him personally and got his calling card and mailed him my published article on Salt Fluoridation in our ACD journal with a personal note asking for his comments on the merits of salt fluoridation in Hawaii. After not hearing from him for two weeks, I called his office to inquire if he got a second copy of the journal from me. He would not even come to the phone or answer my request. I cannot remember his name, but I do remember he was an endodontist. Such behavior of a so-called leader in our profession is not only unacceptable, but also downright rude as well.

Dental Health Work in Armenia

After I read the book by Dr. Estupinan-Day, I wanted to learn more about salt fluoridation for the benefit of the children in the Republic of Armenia. I had traveled to Armenia multiple times with other California Armenian-American dentists to offer humanitarian dental treatment to children in the villages and towns. Armenian children had free dental care during Soviet times, but after the collapse of the Soviet Union and with the establishment of a democratic and capitalistic country, dental care was no longer free for children there. This lack of universal dental care plus a high surgery diet led to a great amount of dental decay among the children. Our dental group was shocked by the large number of cavities in the Armenian children's teeth. We had not seen anything even close in our practices in the U. S.

The implementation of CWF was not feasible because nine reservoirs supplied the water to the mountainous capital city of Yerevan. Therefore, having to implement nine water sources was not economically practical. Besides, most of the agricultural areas had inadequate water facilities.

Since I learned more about the fluoridation options, I concluded that table salt fluoridation was an ideal solution for Yerevan and the rest of the country.

I engaged a public health dentist who actively promoted salt fluoridation in international settings. The ADA recommended Dr. George Gillespie, an English dentist, and he became my mentor. We met online, then when he came to Florida for a vacation, we were together for a week in person. He related his experiences to me. He trained me on how to approach a country in a way that could improve the dental health of its children. He encouraged me to collaborate with the minister of health (MOH) in Armenia to implement salt fluoridation. Later, I brought Dr. Gillespie to the capital city of Yerevan, to meet with the MOH to help me convince the MOH that this form of salt fluoridation was ideal for the prevention of cavities in children. It could be added to iodized table salt. The salts of the two elements, chloride and fluoride, are compatible. Besides, there was an existing salt mine and producer in the country. However, It was necessary to import potassium fluoride or sodium fluoride, along with the required machinery. The existing producer could then integrate one of these two these two micronutrients into the salt. I even hired and brought a consulting salt engineer to Armenia for two weeks. He inspected and approved the existing facilities to be able to implement fluoride in their existing salt. I met five different ministers of health, past and present, over an eight-year period of visiting the country twice a year. Unfortunately, due to bureaucratic red tape, ignorance, corruption, lack of money, and resistance to change, I was not able to implement this dental public health policy in Armenia.

A special World Health Organization (WHO) conference on Oral Health was planned to take place in Geneva in May 2007. The following a year I contacted the MOH in Armenia to urge him to attend this conference. Armenia is also a member of the WHO, and a delegation of two members attended the conference. When I tried to reach our American contingent to introduce them to the Armenian attendees, I was unable to make a connection. At this major conference, the WHO had passed a resolution (WHA.60-17) that salt fluoridation should be used when water fluoridation was not feasible. Despite being a WHO member, the US did not consider policy changes or notify the public about salt fluoridation. Unfortunately, the Armenian MOH and his successors whom I've consulted with never did approve the addition of fluoride to the table salt.

Neither our USPHS nor the CDC has any intention of promoting a way to reach the millions of children who will never have CWF. They continue to follow, I assume, the policy of the ADA that only allows one kind of fluoridation. My guess is that the ADA is still afraid of the antifluoridationists who would demand salt fluoridation be available and that would lead to the discontinuance of CWF.

What are the arguments against the implementation of salt fluoridation as an addition to CWF in the United States? An argument may be made that if children under six years old living in CWF areas also use fluoridated salt, they would get too much fluoride and that may cause fluorosis. The fluorosis that caused the Colorado brown stain is much more severe and unattractive as the natural water in these areas has nine to sixteen parts per million of fluoride. However, there are obvious reasons to rebut both of these arguments.

Fluorosis is not a disease. It is cosmetic coloration of the teeth of children, under six or seven years of age, due to too much fluoride in their diet. Most young people in the US likely have a mild case of this, resulting in white spots on a few front teeth that are not unattractive. To comply with regulations, toothpaste manufacturers must include a warning on all fluoridated toothpaste due to the risk of fluorosis. It states that children under six years of age must be supervised by parents to prevent toothpaste from being swallowed.

In my years in dental school and practice, I have only seen one instance of fluorosis that a dental classmate had. His teeth had a tea-stained color that was plainly observable. However, he never tried to change the way his teeth looked and was happy that he never had any cavities. He was raised in an area where the water contained a high amount of fluoride, such as, 9 to 12 parts of fluoride per million parts of water. Most discoloration issues I have seen of fluorosis are not easily noticed: To see most fluorosis on a patient's teeth, the patient has to be in a dental chair with a dental lamp focused on their teeth.

According to the USPHS report in 2016, more than 90 percent of fluorosis in the United States is the very mild form, most appearing as barely visible lacy-white markings or white spots on the enamel. By comparison, the incidence of fluorosis to the incidence of dental cavities is minuscule. Furthermore, in an article in The Journal of the

American Dental Association in 2013, author Dr. William Bowen concluded that "in most cases fluorosis is a minor cosmetic defect that should not be cause for alarm. Dentists should educate their patients about the optimal range of fluoride intake for caries protection, sources of fluoride and the possibility of fluorosis."

One of my dental students whom I mentored had mild fluorosis on a few of his front teeth, which was hardly noticeable by anyone other than a dentist. I asked him how this happened. He said his mother, who was a dentist, was worried that he might get cavities and was applying fluoride gel frequently to his teeth when he was around six or seven years old.

Dental fluorosis is a minor risk due to too much fluoride in a child's diet from birth to age nine. According to the Food and Nutrition Board of the Institute of Medicine, young people can tolerate the following amounts of fluoride per day without adverse effects: between the ages of four and eight years old, 1.0 mg; from nine to thirteen years of age, 2.0 mg; from fourteen to eighteen years of age, 3.0 mg; and for those ages nineteen years and over, 4.0 mg (https://www.nap.nationalacademies.org/read/5776/chapter/1).

This study by the Institute of Medicine has been ignored by the ADA, USPHS, CDC as they do not recognize the facts that as children mature they can tolerate more fluoride without causing fluorosis. Another argument that may be made is that antifluoridationists would seek to use the efficacy of salt fluoridation to put down CWF. But it is equally true that the parents of children who will never have CWF should have the option to buy table salt with known and proven health benefits for their children—as they do in other countries. Some dentists who are proponents of CWF have said that having salt fluoridation available would give the antifluoridationists another reason to oppose the further implementation of CWF. This is certainly possible.

As I mentioned earlier, salt manufacturers can be required to have labels restricting the use of fluoridated salt in CWF areas. The marketplace will determine where fluoridated salt is available. A supermarket supply buyer would not try to sell a product that restricts usage in their area.

The argument against having two kinds of fluoridation in a country was begun by Dr. Herschel Horowitz. He probably felt children may be exposed to both kinds and have too much fluoride This excessive amount of fluoride in their diet might cause fluorosis of their teeth. Dr. Horowitz was an eminent public health dentist and researcher. He was the lead researcher from America that oversaw the earliest salt fluoridation trials in Antioquia, Columbia. These studies were conducted by the Dental Section of the National Institutes of Health (NIH) during the mid-1960s. The results of these trials provided a clear indication of the beneficial impact of salt fluoridation. Ironically, this research was demonstrated to prove the efficacy of salt fluoridation at US taxpayer expense.

Although I never met the doctor, in 1999, Dr. Horowitz delivered a talk on the national programs of CWF usage, which was followed by the publication of an article on the same topic. At this talk, he stated that a country should only have one kind of fluoridation. However, this talk was presented at a dental school graduation ceremony. This was not a course lecture nor a result of any research. In fact, there has never been any research proving that a country should only have one kind of fluoridation. But that is what he said, and his remarks were published. I found it strange that no one has ever challenged this position, since we are an evidence-based, scientific profession.

In 2012, I proposed a resolution to the House of Delegates, the ruling body of the CDA, to investigate the efficacy of salt fluoridation. The resolution failed. Then in 2013, I proposed another resolution that asked for support of a petition. In this petition, I appealed to the FDA to approve the manufacture and sale of fluoridated table salt. Despite the articles of the efficacy of SF and the resolution passed by the WHO, the FDA denied the petition. This second CDA resolution also failed.

Recently, in December 2024, I proposed yet another resolution to the House of Delegates to "urge the CDA to ask the ADA House of Delegates to investigate and analyze all fluoride containing products for safety, including salt fluoridation." This time, the resolution with amendments, which I accepted, passed unanimously. Hallelujah!

Because the CDA is the largest state component among national chapters, California is known as the bellwether state. It will not be determined until November 2025, in Washington, DC, when the ADA House of Delegates meets again. Stay tuned to the outcome of this resolution.

A reasonable position by the dental profession is to advocate the policy to continue CWF for large communities and implement salt fluoridation as an addition, not an alternative, for small towns that have children on well water. This policy would help children in small towns and rural communities, a population that is more vulnerable to poor dental health. They lack access to free and federally subsidized dental clinics, unlike most children in our major cities.

In addition, why can't the ADA simply advocate and articulate a directive to the public that salt fluoridation can be used for the preventive dental health of children and young adults in locations that do not have CWF? To do this, the ADA must first address the disparity that has come about by the increasing population in non-fluoridated areas. The ADA governance has a House of Delegates, (HOD) that meets annually to consider whatever the membership deems necessary for the improvement of the public's dental health. If they decide that salt fluoridation can be made available along with CWF, I believe the FDA will approve the manufacturer of fluoridated table salt.

I first petitioned the FDA, with a citizen's petition in 2012, to allow the manufacture and sale of fluoridated table salt. The FDA's approval was required for it to be manufactured and sold in the US. However, an approval by the FDA would conflict with the ADA's position on this topic. To support the petition, I referred to the position of the WHO on salt fluoridation. I have also displayed published research articles by Dr. George Gillespie. Gillespie was a public health dentist who helped countries to implement salt fluoridation. Several of my acquaintances supported the petition by emailing their comments. But the ADA and the CDC would not approve nor disapprove of the petition. I am sure they were informed about this petition but chose to ignore it. The ADA and/or the CDC must have some unknown vested interests and stake holders. Perhaps they are afraid that when communities with water fluoridation see that this other type of fluoridation is just as reliable, then they will stop having CWF. In fact, there is an example of this happening: Germany and Mexico had CWF, then ended it and started producing table salt with fluoride.

The petition was denied after two years. I called and spoke to one of the FDA employees to ask why. All he could tell me was that a particular regulation, which I was supposed to look up, was the reason for the denial. This was a typical unsatisfactory bureaucratic answer.

The public would benefit if the FDA and the CDC believed that the dental association knows what is best for the public. There must also be some vested interests that continue to claim CWF, with its obvious limitations, to be adequately reaching our increasingly large population. The facts plainly show that penetration of CWF is diminishing.

Here is an example of the kind of behavior that goes on in our profession on the committee level. Most of these committee people are appointed by the ADA president with input from the regents and other pooh-bahs.

An acquaintance of mine, a dentist from Yakima, Washington, is a member of the ADA Scientific Affairs Committee. I assume some of these committee members are dental researchers. My dentist friend has successfully managed a large subsidized dental clinic for many years that cares for patients who can receive quality care for reduced costs of dental treatment. I had sent him an article I had published in The Journal of the American College of Dentists about the usage of SF in addition to CWF in the U. S. So, I asked him to put salt fluoridation on the agenda at the next meeting to discuss its use where CWF is not available. Sometime after the committee met, I called him back to ask what happened. He replied that the committee did not want to discuss the use of salt fluoridation. No reason was given. This kind of head-in-the-sand decision-making leads me to believe that the ADA and some of their committee members are so bigoted that no one wants to consider or do anything differently for the good of the public they claim to serve.

I am not against CWF, despite its limitations. However, there are professional organizations, other than the ADA, such as the American Academy of Pedodontics Dentistry (AAPD), a specialty group, which should recognize the shortcomings of CWF. They see the ravages of uncontrolled dental cavities daily. I would like to see them step up to the plate and advocate for more than one kind of fluoridation for the sake of children's dental health.

Public policies should aim to support the dental health of all Americans, and I advocate for the approval of salt fluoridation to help the benefits of fluoride reach more American children. It seems strange to me that we can buy fluoridated toothpaste, fluoridated mouthwash, fluoridated supplements, use fluoride gels and fluoridated varnishes, all of which could contribute to fluorosis, if improperly used, but we cannot buy fluoridated salt. Research has been done on these other fluoride products, assessing the risk of fluorosis in areas of CWF among children under six years of age. But no such research exists for the presence of CWF combined with salt fluoridation.

Moreover, there are certainly ethical threads in this anti-salt fluoridation argument. I was trained, like other dental students, to respect patient autonomy and choice, as it is considered part of ethical behavior. Alternate plans of lesser cost or alternate treatment plans are normal approaches to consider the patients' needs. We provide our patients with multiple treatment plans. We should expect no less from our national health agencies and our professional organizations. Let the parents decide on the risk of the two kinds of fluoride available. Especially since the fluoridated salt will have a label limiting its usage to non-fluoridated areas. If we can trust the parents to supervise the use of fluoridated toothpaste with younger children to avoid too much fluoride, why can't we trust them to purchase and use fluoridated salt properly?

Because the dental profession believes in fluoridation as a method to prevent and control dental caries, all means available should be used to improve, by prevention, the dental health of the thirty-eight million American children and young adults in non-fluoridated areas. The time has come for the dental profession to conduct an open debate on the progress and shortcomings of CWF. The issue of using salt fluoridation as an addition to CWF needs to be addressed. There is more than a little evidence that CWF has reached its maximum saturation level in the US population, whether for economic or political reasons, and the reach of

CWF is now losing ground. The cost of CWF is going up with inflation of the cost of specially trained water engineers and the cost of the construction of new water facilities.

Moreover, the backlash against CWF must be recognized and not ignored. The ADA and the AAPD should be able to take a position on this matter. A reasonable position can be taken that CWF is better for large communities and salt fluoridation is better for small towns and children on well water. This position can be supported by the fact that both methods are time-tested and equally effective, as resolved by the WHO. It has been seventeen years since the WHO convened a special meeting on oral health. Plainly, it said that when a country or municipality cannot provide CWF, salt fluoridation is just as efficient to control and prevent dental caries as CWF.

I predict that if the dental profession does not end this disparity in children's dental health, due to only one kind of fluoridation being available, eventually, the informed public will.

The next chapter will discuss dental education with a return to the basics and more ways to better prepare graduates for the practice of dentistry.

4

DENTAL EDUCATION: A RETURN TO THE BASICS

I can tell you from my experience that the worst thing about becoming a dentist was having to go to dental school. Up until the early 1970s, most dental schools, along with medical schools too, were trying to mold students into superman doctors. Most of our full-time faculty were intent on tearing us down and then building us back up to be perfect in every respect. Except they forgot to build us back up again.

What do I mean by saying this? They treated us like military academy plebes. We were not treated like future colleagues. Instead of giving us a compliment for a successful procedure in the laboratory or clinic, we were only criticized for anything less than perfect. Unlike other graduate schools, C, D and F grades could be given. Some of our faculty would threaten us with expulsion. If we received an F grade for any course, we would have to repeat the whole year or be suspended or expelled. Any instructor had that authority.

Every class had one or two students who were repeating the year. This was a constant reminder of what could happen to any of us. In fact, it had a well-known name at my school. It was called the "P & S (physicians and surgeons) merry-go-round." We were trained with a fear of having to repeat the year, or worse, expulsion. Of course, not all the faculty were mean and inconsiderate of our feelings while training us. Many of our volunteers, part-time faculty members, were kind and considerate of the fact that we learned from our mistakes. It is only human to not be able to do something perfectly the first or second time. These faculty members stood out. Not because they were lenient or expected anything less than perfect work, but because they encouraged us to always do our best and become better. They took the time to demonstrate a lab or clinical procedure. Watching someone do something that you are trying to learn to do is called preceptorship. It is an important way of learning. This was the way you became a dentist before there were dental schools. You had an apprenticeship with an experienced dentist.

Fortunately, my school, the University of the Pacific, Dugoni School of Dentistry, started a humanistic program in the mid-1970s, after I graduated, that consisted of treating our students with mutual respect and dignity. In fact, we instructors had to sign a pledge saying that we will treat our students with kindness and consideration —never with harassment or beratement, but as future capable colleagues. In addition, the Commission on Dental Accreditation (CODA) does now require this kind of relationship between student and instructor. When I returned to teaching a dental ethics course in 2003, the students were happy and enthusiastic to be in school learning the skills of becoming a dental surgeon. Our students know that we instructors are there to help them learn in a supportive atmosphere and to become successful graduates. I believe this new model of teaching will have them care for their patients in a more empathetic and compassionate manner.

I do not know if you have ever thought about this, but all dentists must learn to do surgical procedures on patients through what is a 2.5-inch diameter opening of the mouth. For those of you who have never done a surgical procedure in the mouth, it's not an easy thing to learn. Gaining access to the treatment area requires the cooperation of the patient—unlike medical surgery, the patient remains awake the entire time, watching everything you do. And of course, let us not forget that the teeth have the most sensitive nerve structure in the body and must be numbed completely. Just learning how to give a local anesthetic injection, painlessly, is challenging to say the least.

It should be no surprise that dental students are concentrating on learning treatment skills and not thinking or doing anything about prevention. The treatment requirements for graduation do not allow the time to teach dentists how to teach patients how to take care of their teeth and gums. To be a long-lasting success, we dentists know and believe that our treatment is unique in that it requires constant daily maintenance of care and dietary limitations. We must and can do better for our patients by returning to the basics of teaching our patients how to care for their teeth and gums before the restorative treatment they receive.

I am proud of all the accomplishments of the American dental profession. Our treatment and advanced technology are the best in the world. American dentists not only discovered and implemented community water fluoridation to prevent dental decay for children and young adults, but we were also the leaders of implant dentistry for people who have lost one or more of their teeth. As dental students during the 1950s we only dreamed of being able to implant an artificial tooth in the jawbone. This prosthesis can almost replicate a natural tooth perfectly and has become the most popular replacement for a missing tooth.

American dentists started the first dental schools in the world. This happened because medical schools during the 1800s restricted the teaching of dentistry to just one year of the four-year medical school curriculum. The dental graduates of the medical curriculum realized there was much more to learn about how to diagnose and treat the teeth and gums. So, they began dental schools with the curriculum to be four years long. This allowed the inclusion of actual clinical training with patients for the latter two years. This model of training has been adopted worldwide. Moreover, an American dental researcher invented the air-driven turbine drill, which reduced surgical time from hours to minutes; plus, American dental researchers invented many of the dental filling materials and prostheses for replacement of missing teeth.

However, despite all the technological advances of American dentistry, we have not done enough. As I mentioned in chapter 2, most dentists emphasize treatment over prevention even though it is widely known among dentists that 95 percent of dental problems can be preventive. What if you could have fewer treatment appointments because you chose more checkup ones? Wouldn't you be happier going to your dentist? Not to mention the satisfaction you would have from spending less money overall.

There is certainly a problem with the current neglect of emphasizing prevention. One of the solutions to this problem is to tell you about the guiding organization that directs the educational curriculum program of the American dental schools. The American dental school curriculum is under the auspices of the American Dental Association (ADA). The ADA states this: "The dental educational curriculum is a scientifically oriented program which is vigorous and direct intensive." This organization has set certain courses and hours of instruction to maintain the uniform education of dentists across the country. For this purpose, the ADA created the Commission on Dental Accreditation (CODA). Every seven years this agency sends out a team of six dental examiners to visit a dental school for three to four days; the examiners review all the written material of coursework and observe what the students are doing in the clinic and lecture rooms.

The examiners are free to ask anyone, be they staff, students, or instructors, questions about whatever they want answers to. Upon the conclusion of their visit, they meet with department heads to discuss their findings and make recommendations for any changes to the curriculum. The school curriculum committee may be told to strengthen or change some courses. All this data is documented, and a follow-up must be performed by the school showing the changes that they made to their curriculum to become or remain an accredited dental institution. As long as the school teaches the mandatory curriculum, they are complying.

CODA holds semiannual hearings to evaluate and approve new courses that may be adopted by all dental schools. The commission meets in Chicago at the ADA Building to conduct these hearings. An educator or a dentist can submit a new subject or teaching modality for the CODA to review. If the proposal is considered beneficial, hearings are conducted to gather input from educators and other interested parties. If it is approved to be recommended for inclusion in the schools, the person or group who submitted the proposal will be asked to develop the new course. This process takes two or more years to implement for accreditation. Despite the commission's lengthy process of introducing curriculum changes, the schools can make changes in their curriculum on a trial basis without obtaining permission.

As central as Chicago is, the west and east coast dentists must fly to attend these hearings. Given our familiarity with online meetings, why can't hearings be done online? It would save the participants time and money and may also result in having a wider attendance. The CODA director told me that it requires about two years to approve and incorporate a change or addition to the dental school curriculum. I believe that something as important as the education of our dental students ought to be implemented in less than two years.

I have submitted a proposal to the CODA for the revision of predoctoral standards to include dental flossing as being necessary in the education of dental students. In addition, patients should be taught by their dentists to properly floss. I know, firsthand, by talking to my patients and interviewing dentists, that very few, if any, dental professionals teach their patients how to floss properly. It's not possible to learn how to floss correctly by just watching a demonstration, nor by hearing someone explain how to do it, and certainly not by just being told to do it. This skill requires resolute dentist or staff to train patient how to floss properly.

To reach a consensus on the need to teach our dental students how to floss properly, so they can teach their patients, I circulated the following petition to the part-time and full-time faculty members:

Petition to Recommend Basic Oral Hygiene Instructions of Dental Flossing Skills to the Freshmen Class of 2025 and thereafter:

Whereas the dental profession is an evidenced based profession, our Dugoni School of Dentistry claims and assures our students that they are well trained to teach their patients how to prevent periodontal disease, such as, gingivitis.

We members of the Faculty, wish to review and remind the Curriculum Committee of the pivotal research that Dr. Harold Loe did in 1965–66, entitled "Experimental Gingivitis in Man," which proved that gingivitis can be prevented by proper flossing and some brushing within 10–14 days' time. The volunteer subjects had been trained in flossing and had prophylaxis (teeth cleaning) prior to the experiment; thus, proving that bacterial plaque or biofilm, alone, not calculus, causes gingivitis and if not treated may lead to periodontitis. Dr. Loe recorded over 300 different types of bacteria including: cocci, rods, fungi, fusiform and spirochetes in the biofilm. Presently, over 700 bacterial types have been identified, including viruses with the use of an electronic microscope.

Dental and medical scientists now have shown that this biofilm has a direct linkage or may cause these conditions or diseases: low birth weight of newborn, endocarditis, vascular carditis, stroke, diabetes, pneumonia, tonsillitis, middle ear infection and Alzheimer's Disease.

The below listed Faculty members strongly recommend that basic flossing skills be taught to first year students in the Class of 2025, in their Integrated Clinical Science I course; furthermore, that they maintain and have demonstrable excellent periodontal health before progressing to the second year.

Thirty-three faculty members were asked to read this petition without any persuasion on my part. Twenty-nine signed the petition in agreement, the other four did not sign the petition.

Afterward, I request a meeting with the assistant dean and head of the Curriculum Committee. She was a dental hygienist before becoming a dentist and led a dental hygiene school for several years. She called me back and asked if I would mind having the head of the course attend our meeting. I agreed to have him attend. At the meeting a week later, I was instructed to stop circulating the petition, even though neither individual had read it. Their decision was based on information from a few individuals who did not sign. The course head kept telling me that I could not change the curriculum. The students were told to advise the patient to floss but were not shown how. I also mentioned that under the umbrella of academic freedom, I had the right to place my ideas before my fellow faculty members. But finally, I said I would obey their wishes and stop circulating the petition. Besides, my survey proved to me that my fellow instructors agreed on what should be taught to our students. I could not present my findings to the Curriculum Committee.

Later, in a meeting with the dean, I gave him the petition to read and shared the results. Approximately 88 percent of the faculty agreed that the teaching of dental flossing was important to the education of first-year students. The dean sided with the head of the course and the head of the Curriculum Committee. He felt that these two administrators knew better what should be taught than twenty-nine members of his faculty. Naturally, I was sorely disappointed in his decision.

These decision-makers were unaware that our dental students are highly motivated to graduate and will meet any demands. If I asked one of them to do a summersault, the reply would be, "Where should I do it?" The school administration dismissed my petition as worthless or subversive due to its implications for curriculum change.

Real-life experience is essential in dental training for students. Some dental schools have assigned a patient to each student to care for over the entire period of their three- or four-year education. In this way, the student can spend time with their patient like the long-term relationship in a private dental practice. Improving a patient's oral hygiene or dietary habits can take from weeks to years, depending on the dentist's skill and the patient's willingness. Behavior modification or changing unhealthy habits for good ones can influence the patient and the student doctor for the benefit of them both. The student and the patient get to know one another in a more personal way and the student can then effectively see the results of his teaching and treatment. Each dental school has long-term patients who can be attended by multiple students, if needed. Behavior modification can influence the patient and the student doctor for the benefit of them both.

Maintaining both general health and dental health significantly depends on patients adopting better personal hygiene practices and healthier eating habits. Yet there is little or no training of the students in dental schools to teach students how best to help patients to change their habits for better health. When I was a student, we were instructed to ask patients to change their eating and drinking habits, such as drinking diet soft drinks instead of ones with sugar. Or if the patient had a gum chewing or candy habit, to change to nonsugary gum and candies. Training in behavior modification is a reasonable skill to learn in dental school. Often, this advice can help patients to make an informed choice for the better. Still, the best practice is not so simple as asking a patient to change one snack food for another healthier one. Here is an example of behavior modification in a pivotal research project:

Shortly after the research by Dr. Harald Loe proved that gingivitis is caused by bacterial plaque (biofilm) that sticks to the teeth and in the gum cuffs, some dental schools began to have their students replicate his research. My dental school started an experimental gingivitis program among the first-year class. One half of the class would stop flossing and brushing for two weeks. Then the other half would observe the changes in those students' gums as they became irritated, swollen, and easily bleeding. The observing half of the class would then instruct the affected students in proper oral hygiene habits using dental floss and toothbrushing. Within a few days the gum tissues would begin to return to normal health. Then the students switched roles of observers and patients and repeated all steps for two weeks. This teaching method left an indelible impression on the students as their irritated gums returned to normal health upon resuming oral hygiene.

Later, they changed the replication of the original research to having the students just stop brushing and flossing one half of their teeth. This allowed each student to observe the effects of one side of the gum which became inflamed to the other healthier side which stayed healthy with brushing and flossing.

After a few years of teaching students how to control gingivitis, this method was discontinued. I heard a rumor that they stopped this practice because it was deemed inhumane or did not meet Occupational Safety and Health Administration (OSHA) standards. Assuming that this experiment can be done humanely while meeting OSHA requirements, I believe this experimental research should be reintroduced for the training of our students.

Regarding preventing gingivitis among our students, I once asked a fellow course instructor, a periodontist, why we did not teach our students how to floss their own teeth during the first year. He replied saying that "they would pick it up along the way." This was during a course teaching our students how to diagnose gum disease and the use of periodontal instruments. Since I had the experience of teaching my own patients how to use dental floss, I can tell you that learning how to use floss in your own mouth was just as challenging and difficult as learning to use some of our dental instruments. Moreover, patients are more likely to be convinced if the student doctor is practicing what he preaches.

Later, we expected our students to demonstrate the usage of these various dental instruments. Evaluating the students for their ability to use the instruments properly is necessary. So is assessing a student's ability to use dental floss. In the school's dental hygiene program, students are taught how to effectively use dental floss and are supervised to ensure they become proficient in this skill. Should the education of a dental student cover fewer topics than that of a dental hygienist? I do not think so.

It is absurd that dental students receive less training

in dental floss use than dental hygienists. In the hands of a dental student, hygienist, or dentist, floss is an instrument. All instrument usage requires training and practice.

Regarding where and when dentists learned to floss, I interviewed thirty dentists who had attended different dental schools throughout the country, from coast to coast. Only one dentist reported receiving instruction on how to floss their teeth in school. Additionally, they were required to demonstrate this essential home care procedure. They advised patients to floss to prevent disease. I believe to change and improve patient behavior; dentists must practice what they preach. They must be a shining example of good dental health maintained by excellent oral hygiene habits.

In school, dental students will learn whatever they think or are told what will be on their examinations. If students are not evaluated on a subject or technique, they do not feel it is important to learn. We learn in many ways, such as, from listening to lectures, reading, and observing. But the best learning comes from doing it under supervision and repetition of practicing. The dental curriculum should include skills for flossing and teaching patients how to floss.

Although a great deal of research has been done in the past on teeth diseases, it was not until the 1950s and 1960s that research was done, using the electron microscope, of gingival tissues or gums. This research investigated the diverse types of bacteria found surrounding the tooth and spaces between the teeth. Not only were there specific bacteria identified that are associated with periodontal diseases, but all types of other organisms that can affect one's general well-being.

Here is how this bacterial plaque works to cause gum irritation and bleeding. The bacterial plaque (biofilm), in the gum cuff space around each tooth, sticks to our teeth. Five hundred to seven hundred diverse types of bacteria make up the oral microbiome. This microbiome colonizes and increases in population after a few days and becomes more virulent than any one single bacteria. When these diverse kinds of bacteria interact, they can colonize and proliferate to form a more virulent combined strain. Some of the various bacterial organisms include cocci and bacterial rods, viruses, fusiform, fungi, and even spirochetes. This microbiome (biofilm) causes inflammation of the gum tissues. Thus, it is the toxic chemicals or poisons of inflammation that break down the thin tissue barrier and that lead to bleeding and entry of bacteria into the bloodstream. Once these toxic irritants are removed or disrupted for five to ten consecutive days, the healing tissues restore the thin skin barrier and the bleeding stops. The gums return to normal. Fortunately, our gingival tissues are the second most regenerative tissues in the body.

When our gums show signs of inflammation or gingivitis, it is the precursor of periodontitis. The medical profession now recognizes that inflammation of the gums is a contributory factor in many medical diseases. It was first noted with an association of low birth weight of infants and mothers who have gingivitis or periodontitis during pregnancy. Then cardiac surgeons discovered P. gingivalis, the primary bacteria in periodontitis, in the diseased heart valves of patients with inflammation (endocarditis). Today, cardiac and vascular surgeons and some cardiologists require a dental checkup to assure them that the gums are healthy and not inflamed before performing heart surgery or invasive vascular procedures. Some other medical diseases that are linked to gum inflammation are the following: diabetes, metabolic syndrome, cardiovascular disease, stroke, pneumonia, tonsillitis, otitis media, and Alzheimer's disease.

I have treated numerous patients with inflamed or bleeding gums. I assigned my dental therapist to teach my patient how to floss their teeth over a month's time with seven to eight thirty-minute appointments. These appointments started with five consecutive days followed by one or two the next week, and then an additional checkup in a month. I promised my patients that their gums would stop bleeding in ten to fourteen days. Oftentimes, whether calculus is present or not, mechanical abrasion by toothbrushing the outer gum tissues and scraping in between the teeth with dental floss or other devices will remove or disrupt the causative irritation of biofilm.

Rinsing your mouth with mouthwash or using an oral irrigator will not remove the sticky substance of the biofilm. These products and rinsing only remove loose food particles. Despite the advertisements you hear and see on television for the prevention of gum disease, they are false and not scientifically proven. They are not based on evidence from research. One popular mouthwash claim that it removes the plaque above the gum better than flossing. Of course, but that is not what flossing is for. Plaque below the gum or around the tooth is more important than plaque above the gum. The plaque on the teeth is easily removed with toothbrushing.

Just as important as having the know-how to educate the patient is to have the conversational ability to communicate with the patient. What I have observed over the course of teaching dental students is that successful students are the ones that have developed good conversational skills. The students that come to us with these attributes are the ones that do better right from the start. Teaching conversational skills has to be a part of the curriculum for some of the students. Dentistry depends on talking to patients to gain their confidence and trust to convince them to change and adopt better oral hygiene and dietary habits.

I was surprised by my full-denture professor of prosthetics, Dr. Jack Werner, when he required us to read Dale Carnegie's classic book How to Win Friends and Influence People. At that time, my classmates laughed at this requirement and made jokes about the need to read it. Later, after we completed the fabrication of the full denture teeth and gave patients their new teeth, we realized the need to build a friendly relationship with our patients. Now we had to convince and persuade our patients to wear and use what we made for them to eat with. Imagine trying to teach someone how to use an artificial leg to walk with it and then teach them how to dance with it. Getting a patient to learn to talk and eat with their new dentures is just as difficult.

Along with learning how to communicate well with patients, many dental students who arrive in dental school would benefit from learning the wisdom of "Physician (or in this case, Dentist), heal thyself." When dental students come to school having the same gum problems that many of our patients have, this presents a teaching moment.

Forming these habits requires training and practice to adopt and retain as lifelong habits. I think it is strange that our students are not expected to graduate with good dental health and nutritional habits. One may argue that our students are legal adults and entitled to monitor their own lifestyles. However, there are still rules we need to enforce and good decisions we can advise them to make regarding their personal habits.

Here are of the rules of behavior and advice that the students at my school receive and in some cases, must obey:

- No smoking in or around the school building.
- Get a roommate to live with close by, unless you are married. It helps to have a study partner or group.
- Avoid illegal drug usage. Addiction to any substance must be avoided.
- Consider engaging in team sports for maintaining a level of physical fitness.
- Don't bring a car, motorcycle, or bike to school. It will only be a liability in San Francisco due to parking and traffic conditions.
- Avoid snacks with high sugar content. We eliminated the soft drink vending machines due to the sugar content.
- Obtain the free vaccinations on premises for the flu and COVID-19. It is mandatory that all students have the required hepatitis B vaccination and other vaccinations. (This is state law handed down to healthcare personnel.)
- Dress properly for classes, the lab, and the clinic, as this is mandatory.
- Properly groomed hair and beard are mandatory in the clinic.

Finally, we employ a nurse and psychologist to be available at school for any student who may wish to consult with them regarding their general and emotional health. In the nurse's reception room, on a coffee table, there is a bowl of condoms. Now, with all these rules, advice, and expectations of our students regarding their behavior and lifestyle, shouldn't they be expected to have excellent dental health during and after their education?

The ideal education of a healthy professional person should not end with the training and treatment of the patient. It must result in a calling for the student doctors to change their lifestyles as well. Moreover, the true professional person must be, in effect, a lifelong, continuous student to provide the best care for patients. As discussed earlier, changes or new treatment modalities start in the private dental offices long before the schools incorporate new treatments. When new instruments are designed or new materials are invented or new research findings become evident, changes in school curriculum and training must occur.

Fortunately, many American dentists form and join study clubs. They come together to learn and share knowledge from each other about new materials and instruments or to discuss research findings to improve their treatment for their patients. The main guiding principle is that of who has the "best practices." This concept of best practices should be recognized within the faculties of our schools that have part-time dental practitioners who teach. They can introduce needed changes that can help the schools to better prepare the students for practice outside of school.

After completing dental school, dentists continue their education to stay updated with recent technological advancements. I was active in The Academy of General Dentistry, which was instrumental in establishing the regulations regarding continuing education (CE) for dentists in California. After they complete formal dental education, all dentists are required by their state to keep up with continuing their education due to the advances in dental technology and research. The Dental Board of California requires fifty hours of CE every two years to renew one's dental license. In fact, the dental profession was one of the earliest professions to establish CE as a mandatory requirement for licensure renewal in California.

Our CE courses are available online and in lectures and courses at local, regional, statewide or national dental meetings, as well as at dental schools. It is at these meetings that dentists can hear about new medicines, materials, techniques, and research to better care for their patients. The dental schools do not usually have this kind of information in their undergraduate curriculum. This is not to say that faculty members are unaware of this new knowledge. But the school curriculum is not constantly changing immediately to include the most up-to-date information. Dental school instruction and teachings are conservative. New techniques are introduced into dental education several years subsequent to their initial adoption by practicing dentists.

For instance, as a private practicing dentist, along with other dentists, I started doing implant dentistry after taking a 40-hour CE course many years after graduation and long before it was taught in dental schools. Our technology is constantly changing, and CE allows us to keep up with the advancements in our profession.

More recently, I took a course about the importance and detection of biofilm that I wish my students could see and hear. This course used a phase-contrast microscope to look at the tooth biofilm of a patient. It was not just very revealing, but shocking. The advantage of this kind of microscope is not just magnifying the biofilm that sticks to our teeth in the gum crevices around the tooth. It also allows the operator to take the patient's specimen and directly place it on the viewing platform, without any need for staining, and instantly see the various kinds of bacteria swimming around. Believe me, if you saw these live bacterial organisms from your mouth under the microscope, you would not want to go to bed without flossing your teeth to get rid of them.

Some dental offices have these microscopes so that they can motivate their patients to disrupt and remove biofilm daily to prevent inflammation of the gums. Our school has several types of microscopes; one or two are phase-contrast microscopes but are located far away from the clinic in a laboratory. So, they are not easily available to image patient specimens. Relocating the scopes would not be difficult. All that would remain necessary would be teaching students how to use the microscope. The demonstration of showing patients what is going on in their mouths helps patients to be more motivated to improve their oral hygiene.

I'll finish the chapter with some takeaway points I feel are important regarding the education of dentists. First, the emphasis of their training should be on preventing tooth and gum disease by teaching the students that most dental treatment is subject to failure. They should understand that dental treatment only gives our patients a second chance to avoid decay and the recurrence of inflammation of the gums.

Secondly, first-year students should learn how to maintain and have excellent dental health before advancing to the second year of training. They should also have access to a phase-contrast microscope in the clinic to reveal the living bacteria in biofilm for educating themselves and for their patients.

Another inclusion in the curriculum should be a course on nutritional science. After all, just because you teach a patient how to maintain excellent oral hygiene habits does not mean dental decay will be stopped. It is imperative for our students to have knowledge of all the foods containing hidden sugar. Learning to eat more healthy whole foods has a paramount influence on our dental and medical health.

Finally, a course on patient-behavior modification of oral hygiene and dietary habits should be added to the curriculum. Again, the establishment of a trusting relationship between the patient and the doctor must precede any change in behavior. I believe that the inclusion of these courses in dental education will better train dentists to be more successful in helping their patients become independently healthy to prevent the continuation of the oral disease processes.

Even though dentists receive extensive education and ongoing training, dental insurance companies often ignore new treatment advances through their fee allowance tables. The next chapter will cover the role of dental insurance companies and their impact on treatment.

5

DENTAL INSURANCE PLANS

Dental insurance is not really a form of insurance in the normal sense of the word. It is more a form of prepaid dental care. The reason being that to prevent dental disease, which can be detected earlier than most other medical problems, it is advisable to have checkups once or twice a year. Dental insurance is not the typical form of medical insurance that will prevent you from having a costly medical surgery or hospital stay. It is just prepaying predictable expenses for periodic checkups and preventive procedures to avoid more costly treatment. Despite these limitations, it is now regarded as the most highly valued benefit in an employer's compensation package.

Many visit the dentist simply because they have dental insurance. Dental insurance has certainly increased the frequency of patients seeking dental care since its inception in the late 1950s. However, very few patients know what their policy is going to pay for and who they may have to go to for dental care. Regardless of these drawbacks, there has been greater access to dental care due to dental insurance. Today, people are keeping their teeth longer, and the need for complete full dentures is reduced. A significant portion of the interest and demand for dental care can be attributed, in part, to the availability of dental insurance.

Even though more people are keeping their natural dentition now, it is estimated that forty million Americans between the ages of sixty-five and seventy-four are missing most or all of their teeth. Patients want dental care, not only to avoid tooth loss, but to maintain an attractive smile, partly because it is a benefit of their employment compensation. While dental insurance companies have been a benefit to millions of people, they have not kept up with increasing dental costs or advances in dental treatment. The fee-allowance tables of procedures are archaic. These tables list payments for fees that the insurance companies are willing to pay. Typically, they are lower than dentists' usual, customary, and reasonable fees (UCR).

These tables were set up in the early 1960s. Fifty-four years later, the yearly allowance barely covers partial treatment for a patient who has not seen a dentist in years. The insurance companies have not raised their fees or the maximum allowance per year. For instance, the maximum payment for an entire year is fifteen hundred dollars ($1,500). This dollar amount would allow a patient to have one or two teeth cleanings or a couple of fillings. The expense of a crown would be partially covered, accounting for 25 percent of the costs after the copayment and the 50 percent allowance on prosthetic-care procedures.

Furthermore, the allowable procedures are plainly outdated and usually do not cover oral hygiene instructions (OHI) that are paramount to maintaining the dental treatment that a dentist has done. Dental insurers can exclude procedures beneficial to patients. If OHI is covered, only one session is permitted per year, despite proper flossing instruction requiring four to eight sessions over several weeks.

Unfortunately, people with employer-paid dental insurance do not regularly go for well-patient dental care. The insurance companies love these kinds of patients— they are laughing all the way to the bank. Employee usage of dental insurance policies is only about 60 percent. During COVID, it was even less, as patients were afraid to see their dentist, thinking they may expose themselves to the COVID virus.

So, 40 percent of insured patients do not go to the dentist annually for checkups. This group of people only go when they have a painful toothache or when they notice bleeding gums.

The traditional forms of dental insurance are more like an indemnity insurance policy which guarantees you against injury, loss, or damage. In other words, you go to your dentist of choice or one that a friend recommended, and your treatment is based on the insurance company's table of allowed procedures. The insurance company would designate a percentage of payment toward that type of treatment. For example, for the initial examination, cleaning, a few X-rays, or a filling, the insurance company would pay 100 percent. But for more complicated treatments, such as crowns or replacement of teeth, they would possibly pay just 50 percent of the dentist's fees. The dentist would charge his usual, customary, and reasonable (UCR) fee. In most cases, the patient will then assign the insurance payment to the dentist and pay a copayment charge to the dentist to initiate the treatment. Upon satisfactory completion of the treatment, the dentist will receive payment from the insurance company. Most private practice dentists accept these kinds of insurance to work with.

Many patients do not fully understand the several types of plans available today. They are not like the traditional type of indemnity plans. Most patients need the dental staff to explain what their dental coverage is for various types of procedures. In my private dental practice, my receptionist had the details of about forty to fifty insurance companies with a total of up to 400 different plans available among these companies. Without a computer it would have been impossible to keep track of what plans a patient might have. Besides the two types of insurance plans, one similar to an indemnity insurance policy, and the other one which has a table of what fees the insurance company would pay for, there are now other types of plans that are available. Most state regulations allow the dental insurance industry to offer health maintenance organization (HMO) and preferred provider organization (PPO) types of plans.

These HMOs and PPOs can make contracts directly with dentists to do the insurance company's bidding. What do I mean by that? Some insurance companies enlist twenty to thirty dentists in a local area or town to form a network of dental providers. Your own family dentist is often not on the network, so you cannot go to your own family dentist and get coverage from these plans. Or if you go to your own dentist, the covered fee, or fee allowance, will be a lowered amount of payment.

Once HMOs or PPOs form their networks, they send each of these dentists about 300 to 500 patients. The insurance companies pay the dentists very little each month for each of these potential patients, whether or not the patient receives treatment. The dentist is required to perform almost all necessary treatments for the patient, with no other compensation. If prosthetic treatment, the one exception, is needed, the insurance company determines what the dentist can charge the patient. Imagine having to work under these financial conditions.

Of note, the treatment procedures in these networks are limited and the fees paid are below the UCR that the contracted dentist charges other patients.

Many times, I was asked to enroll in these types of plans, as were my dental colleagues who were established or had been in practice for five or more years. We could see the pitfalls and ethical compromise that would result from this way of conducting a private dental practice. My dental friends and I never signed these kinds of business contracts. They were not in either the patient's best interest or the interest of the dentist.

There are several reasons why I say this. To begin with, the Dental Practice Act in California and similar acts in many other states have laws against "capping and steering" of individuals. Before there were state laws and regulations for dentists and physicians, some doctors in the late 1800s and early 1900s would hire a person to find a patient with a dental or medical problem and bring them to the doctor's office. This "capper" would receive a payment for "steering" the patient to the doctor. The doctor would then add the cost of the capper to the patient's fee for their treatment. This obviously underhanded practice was and still is illegal. Now, this form of practice is legalized by most states for dental insurance corporations, but it is still illegal for individual dentists to do. If patients and employee-benefits managers knew the facts, they would not select these types of so-called dental insurance plans. They are chosen due to their cost-effectiveness compared to other indemnity dental plans available.

The young dentists who need to be busier sign up for these kinds of plans. The more established dentists realize that these plans are a financial risk, and they do not go into these kinds of contracts with the insurance companies.

In my mind, there is not much difference between these HMO dental insurance policies with capitation and the illegal practice for doctors to hire someone to send them patients. In both cases the patients are steered to a group of dentists who are paying a go-between by lowering their fees and giving the insurance company a profit. Although these types of dental insurance plans are legal, I still question their ethics.

If the patients really understood that their doctor is at risk of not doing the best treatment or a needed treatment for them due to financial constraints of such capitation plans, they would want another doctor who puts his patients' interest first. Health professionals should be able to be financially secure. There should not be a conflict between prioritizing patients' needs and the ability for a healthcare professional to earn a living.

HMOs and PPOs also limit the patient's choice of dentist or physician, as the insurance company determines the selection. You might give up your freedom of choice to keep a doctor whom you have a trusting relationship with for some unknown person. When your doctor knows you and your dental condition, this personal relationship leads to the best care possible.

To give you an example, one of my longtime elderly dental patients told me she was always pleased with my dental care. However, her husband chose another type of dental insurance plan with a network of dentists that she would have to choose between to go to. She asked if I would kindly look at a list of the plan's dentists and select the best one for her to go to. I said that I would look at the list but wanted to get my San Francisco Dental Society directory for comparison. At that time, about 900 of approximately 1,200 dentists belonged to the SF Dental Society. I got out the SFDS directory and sat down with her to look at the list of about thirty network dentists. I went over her list twice and did not see any of these network dentists belonging to the dental society. So, I told her that I could not recommend any of them. She was surprised and asked what difference that made. I told her that the members of the SFDS had higher ethical standards than dentists who did not belong to the group. Furthermore, if a patient was displeased with the dental care they received, they could file a complaint with the dental society peer review committee. All our members are subject to peer review by other members on the committee. Furthermore, 70 percent of the time they rule in favor of the patient. So, I told her I was sorry that I could not recommend any of the network dentists even though they had a license to practice. I also said the best care is with someone that is not just legally qualified, but practices ethically as well.

HMOs and PPOs that contract the dentist are a bad choice for dentists to sign up for because they place the dentist in a difficult position. Consider the fact that before most dentists sign up for these plans, they have a number of private patients who pay their UCR fees. These dentists are required to treat patients for whom they receive compensation that is below the UCR fees for identical treatments and laboratory costs. Which patients are going to receive the dentist's best effort and care? When the dentist has a difficult procedure or difficult patient, who is going to receive the best treatment? Will it be the patient who is paying the full fees or the one for whom the dentist receives less than the full fees? Which patients will be reminded of periodic checkup appointments? It becomes clear how these plans can compromise a dentist's treatment and care.

But what is even more compromising are dental service organizations, such as HMO dental plans that pay the dentist a monthly fee for each patient, whether the patient comes to the office for treatment or not. These were referred to earlier, and are called capitation plans, wherein the dentist receives a monthly payment of about six to eight dollars per patient for a roster of 400 to 500 assigned patients. The dentist is then obliged to do all the emergency and routine treatment, such as cleanings, X-rays, fillings, and extractions for no charges at all and/or a copayment. Then if the patient needs crowns, bridges, or partial or full dentures, the dentist must charge less than their usual fees and collect a copayment from the patient. The dentist has no prior information on what some of the patient's treatment needs may be and must do all the dental care needed.

Imagine, if you were the dentist and that month the cost of treatment you did for patient on the capitation plan already exceeded what you were paid for that month. How interested would you be in seeing and giving appointments to more of these capitation insured patients? In these plans the dentist is financially at risk and compromised. The doctor can just put off other patients who need treatment now to a later time. The state dental association can try to educate the young dentists, but they cannot say that these plans are a bad deal and advise young dentists not to sign up or enter contracts with them. If they did this, they would be liable for a lawsuit.

This is not to say all dental insurance plans are not worth the paper they are written on. The traditional indemnity plans can certainly save you some money. But as good as the indemnity dental insurance plans are, they do limit dental procedures that are important for patients to have. One such example is a night guard splint. Let's look at that example.

Some patients unknowingly grind or clench their teeth while sleeping. This habit is called bruxism and can lead to several symptoms and diseases. To begin with, these patients usually complain of morning headaches, painful or tired jaws, and/or teeth sensitivity. Sometimes, the dentist can observe and show the patient that they have been doing this habit for a long time. There may be wear (facets) on their back teeth that are demonstrable.

Bruxism can be very destructive, causing several more problems. As a result of grinding, oftentimes the teeth can fracture, gums may recede, teeth become loose, or the nerve of a tooth can become infected. Very few of these symptoms or problems can be seen on an X-ray until it is too late. And yet, many insurance companies usually do not include dental guard coverage, a treatment that can eliminate pain and disease and save teeth from loss. Insurance companies do not care whether or not you maintain good dental health. They care more about making sure their "dental loss ratio" (DLR) is small compared to their gross profit margin. The DLR is the cost that the insurance company pays out to the dentist for a patient's care. The rest is their profit margin. Although having dental insurance benefits encourage people to get dental checkups and treatment, not all the policies are designed in the interest of the patient.

Sad to say, the HMOs and PPOs are part of the dental marketplace. These are the types of dental insurance plans that are being purchased for the employees, but not for the executives of the companies. The plans of company executives have been like the traditional ones that include almost all procedures, such as orthodontics and implants, with little or no copayments. I recommend that you complain to your employee-benefits manager. Tell them you want the traditional indemnity dental plans that allow you to go to the dentist of your choice.

As a buyer of dental insurance, I am recommending you employ caveat emptor, that is, "buyer beware." Yes, dental insurance of the indemnity type can reduce your dental treatment costs. But I believe that the best dental care can be achieved when there is no one or no entity between the patient and the doctor, whether you are seeking dental care or medical care. I say this because anyone else involved in your care complicates and sometimes compromises your personal health care.

Fortunately, there is a dental care payment program that allows you to select your own dentist and have your employer help pay for some or all of your care without compromise and complications. These plans are called direct payment dental plans. Tell your benefits manager to look it up at the California Dental Association website, https://www.cda.org. Other states may also offer this kind of plan too. This type of insurance payment goes directly to the cost of your dental care with no "middleman" or insurance company receiving part of the money.

Here is the straightforward way it works: If, for example, your employer is willing to allow reimbursement of $1,000 per year for your dental care, you simply present your employer benefit manager the receipt of your completed dental treatment or the estimated amount. Payment is then directly paid to you or your dentist of choice. Thereby, you have avoided a table of allowed dental procedures, and all your reimbursed services go directly to the actual cost of the treatment. Direct payment allows you to continue with the dentist you know and trust or have the freedom to choose whomever you want to go to.

While the private sector has created dental corporations for folks with or without dental insurance coverage, the federal government is on the brink of including dental care for Medicare patients. However, until dental care becomes allowable in the Medicare health program for seniors, it will not be recognized by our government as being an important aspect of health care. Each year legislative bills are introduced in Congress that allow dental care of certain Medicaid patients. The ADA is now interested in some level of participation. This is a first step in the direction of making dental care a part of Medicare for some or all the participants.

It is just a matter of time before Medicare will include participants with dental care services that want them. I believe that the main reason for keeping this aspect of health care coverage from becoming a reality is the future cost. It is difficult to determine how costly dental care may become as there are many seniors over sixty-five who are edentulous (have no natural teeth). This number is estimated to be around 10 percent of the Medicare recipients.

The costliest treatment for seniors is the replacement of teeth, or prosthetic dental care. One of the ways to reduce the cost is to request copayment by the participants. I have always felt that our Medicare program should have copayments.. This feature would reduce the cost, but not without raising the cost of Medicare to working salaried folks and their employers.

Another way to reduce the cost of Medicare with dental services is to allow participants to have the option to opt out of dental care insurance. The folks that want dental services could have a choice between different levels of dental plans, such as HMOs or PPOs. In this way, the people that can afford to go to their private dentist of choice will not be charged for services they do not wish. This is the same way Medicare patients have a choice of different levels of drug insurance plans or can just pay for their prescription out of pocket. Patients should have the freedom to choose their own doctors and surgeons.

I believe that the dental profession is now ready to accept Medicare patients if the overhead cost of dental services is recognized as being greater than in office medical services. The dentists must receive a reasonable profit. After all, all dentists are surgeons working in private-office settings that have costly equipment and instruments and must maintain hospital standards of sterilization.

Fortunately, most private practice dentists do not get into contracts with insurance companies that market the HMOs and PPOs that are cheaper for employers to buy. These plans are adopted by federally subsidized clinics because they are much cheaper than the indemnity types of dental insurance policies.

But not everyone needs dental insurance. For many years, before dental insurance was available, people used to pay their doctors out of pocket. Back then, many dentists and physicians would accommodate their patients in need, by reducing their charges for folks that couldn't afford the full fee for the services. Today, the government has made it easy for you to save up money to have dental or medical care. It is called the health savings account (HSA). Moreover, the money you set aside for your health services is treated like pension plan money; it is not taxed. This is an ideal way for you to have the funds saved to pay for your dental care, if you don't have dental insurance. I recommend that an HSA be used with or without dental insurance as this savings account can be used for most any dental or medical expenditure that may be necessary. It can also be used to pay for any health insurance premium that you may have.

The dental plans provided by employers are group plans. For individuals, there are individual dental insurance policies. I have investigated them and studied the costs of individual dental insurance policies, but I do not recommend them for most folks. The individual dental insurance plans cost more per year than you would normally pay without any insurance. If you usually have a dental examination, cleaning, and occasional X-rays, once or twice each year, with no further need for treatment, I recommend simply paying for this preventive care out of pocket. You can go to whomever you want for your dental care and stay with the dentist that you have a trusting relationship with. This can be your best care without needing to go to a dentist on an insurance company list.

On the other hand, if you know that you need a crown or have missing teeth that could be replaced with a partial denture, bridge, or implant, don't think you can outsmart the dental insurance companies' individual plans. These plans have clauses in them that do not allow an existing condition to be treated until you have spent one year on the plan—or not at all. If you feel you can wait a year and then have the more costly procedures done, the percentage they pay for a preexisting condition is very small. It is very difficult or impossible to game or outsmart these companies.

If you choose to eliminate a third-party payer, such as an insurance plan, to try and reduce your dental costs, it's good to know most dentists accept credit or debit card payment. But if your dental costs are greater than your savings or cash on hand, most dental offices also have special payment plans that are less costly than the credit card companies' interest charges. In fact, some of these healthcare credit plan payment companies, which you may qualify for, allow you to have them pay your dental bill and you receive the dental care that you need. Oftentimes, there is no interest charge if you pay back the borrowed amount within four to six months.

In summary, the dental marketplace today presents a real dilemma for dental patients. The days of going to your family dentist or the dentist of your choice may be gone. Many working people are given dental insurance plans that do not allow them to go back to their family dentist. These plans can save you some money, but you must research what kind of plan you have. If you can afford to select your own dentist from among the available plans, I believe you will receive the best care.

In my experience, the HMO and PPO insurance plans do not attract the best dentists in the community. Take the time to research the list of network dentists by making an appointment to have the receptionist or office manager explain the limitations of the insurance plan that you have, in person, before you make an appointment for any treatment. If they are unwilling, try another office.

Or simply call your local dental society for a dentist member that is known for doing preventive dental care. Ask the dental office personnel if they can teach you how to floss properly and the details of the program. You can also ask your friends if they recommend their dentist and pick the dentist who is held in the highest regard. Finding the dentist that helps you to prevent dental diseases will give you the personal attention you deserve and is worth the time and money spent.

In the next chapter, I will discuss nontraditional dental offices that have come into existence through the federal government. These clinics accommodate the needs of children and adults who live in communities that do not have private dental offices and accommodate those who feel they cannot afford to have care in private dental offices.

6

SUBSIDIZED DENTAL CLINICS

Federally Qualified Health Centers (FQHC) are a safety net that can provide dental care to uninsured patients or patients with dental insurance. It also covers people with Medicare and Medicaid or Denti Cal as it is called in California.

Dental care is becoming recognized as an essential part of the services of the Centers for Medicare and Medicaid Services (CMS). According to the American Academy of Periodontists, half of all Medicare beneficiaries, about twenty-four million people, don't have dental insurance. And it is estimated that two-thirds of these folks suffer from periodontal disease. The US Senate issued a letter urging the CMS to expand dental coverage for better general health. It should be no surprise that the US Centers for Medicare and Medicaid

Services (CMS) has proposed a rule to expand dental coverage under Medicare. Therefore, sixteen million Medicare patients that have some degree of gum disease may adversely affect their general health. As these folks are all over the age of sixty-six years old, this gum infection can be the nidus of bacteria streaming through their blood vessels, causing the artery walls to thicken, reducing the lumen or diameter, and initiating hypertension.

These health care centers for adults and children must provide comprehensive, high-quality, and culturally competent services. They are often located in neighborhoods and communities experiencing poverty and with insufficient access to primary care. In addition, most major cities have clinics for school children under the Medicaid programs.

In San Francisco, there are five dental clinics located in neighborhoods experiencing poverty to accommodate the dental needs of children living in these districts. The reason some children in these districts do not receive early care is that the child must be accompanied by a parent or an adult caregiver. When both parents work or are not aware of the importance of early preventive care, the child suffers. These clinics also offer services to women who are pregnant. The lack of dental care of the gums during pregnancy can cause low-birth weight deliveries or preterm delivery.

I was personally involved with the passage of a law to add dental examinations to the existing requirement for eye and hearing examinations for children entering public schools. In California, all school children, including those in kindergarten, now must have a dental screening examination showing no need for any dental care in order to enroll as a student. If treatment is necessary, the parents must seek care for their child before being admitted to schooling.

Here is part of the background leading to my involvement in establishing the requirement for children's screening examinations without X-rays. The California Dental Association (CDA) wanted to have dental examinations added to the requirement in addition to hearing and eyesight examinations for public school education.

One morning, on my way to my office at 450 Sutter Street in San Francisco, Mayor George Moscone entered the elevator that I was in. After a few people got off, we were the only ones in the elevator. I introduced myself and told the mayor that I was in Sacramento earlier that month for Doctor's Day at the Capital. I told him I was disappointed that the state senators did not understand that we should direct the limited amount of Denti-Cal funds to emergencies for adults. The state should concentrate on the children's preventive health programs, I shared, so the children grow up with fewer dental problems than their parents. Also of note is the fact that treatment services for adults are more costly than the preventive services for children. Mayor Moscone agreed with me that what we dentists had recommended made better sense. But, as he left the elevator he said, "Unfortunately, the children can't vote." So that is the way it goes.

It took almost ten years to convince the legislature of the importance of this dental screening examination for children's health and well-being. The legislators claimed that the dentists were trying to promote their business and increase their income with more patients. The dentists belonging to the CDA finally convinced the legislature by having the state dental association declare that the association member dentists would do this examination for any child at no cost. We had to inform the parents if treatment was needed. The parents could then seek dental care wherever they wanted.

Presently, the San Francisco-based children's dental health clinics employ dental hygienists to canvas the schools and perform the children's screening examinations. The hygienists can issue a dental report form to each child's parent indicating the needs and where to take a child if they do not have a family dentist.

This way of employing hygienists in public schools makes a lot of sense. The hygienist's skills and training are too valuable and extensive to restrict them to just cleaning and polishing children's teeth in the office setting of these city clinics. It is also a way to identify a child's dental needs if they have not returned to the clinic for semiannual checkups.

Unfortunately, these clinics only perform treatment based on dental insurance tables of allowed procedures of the patient's dental insurance plan. Or the table of allowances of the Medicaid program. These tables do not permit oral hygiene instruction. If OHI is allowed, it is only once each year. A child or an adult cannot learn how to take proper care of their teeth with a single appointment once a year.

Moreover, the treatment done for children, once or twice a year, is a cleaning of their teeth. An examination with back-teeth X-rays is also done to detect cavities between the teeth that the dentist cannot easily see. Most children don't need to have their teeth cleaned. Polishing is usually done but does not have as much value as teaching the child how to clean their teeth at home. This training of proper use of dental floss and a toothbrush can help to make the child independently healthy. In other words, current visits to these clinics are based on treatment, not prevention.

Besides federally subsidized clinics offering dental services to the public, there are now dental corporations that offer dental services. This subject will be discussed in the next chapter.

7

THE RISE OF CORPORATE DENTISTRY

Corporate dentistry is the formation of salaried dentists and supportive auxiliaries, such as bookkeepers, receptionists, hygienists, and dental assistants, working for a corporation that provides dental care to patients for a profit. According to new data, 13 percent of dentists nationwide are affiliated with a dental service organization. Their popularity among recently graduated dentists, less than ten years out of school, is much higher.

A dental corporation can be established by buying dental practices that are for sale and hiring one of the former owners to continue as a salaried senior manager in the corporation.

Of course, dentistry has always had a commercial aspect to it, as all dental practices must practice good monetary management to stay operational. But corporate dentistry is making sure that the bottom line has a margin of profit for the company shareholders, in addition to paying the dentist and staff salaries. Since this type of dental practice is relatively new, it remains to be seen how successful this type of dental practice will be.

The business aspects of dentistry are covered and discussed in dental schools under the topic of Practice Management. However, most courses are not more than 10 lecture-hours long, and they do not adequately prepare the new graduate dentist with enough know-how to properly conduct a private practice.

For instance, I was trained in dental school to not only present my treatment plan to my patient, but to make financial arrangements with the patient directly. Most patients needed more time to pay for their services than the time needed to do the treatment. We had to repay the school if the patient could not cover the services. So, we learned how to manage that risk by establishing a financial plan with the patient before performing our services. Nowadays, most dental schools have financial clerks to make payment plans with patients. Unless the graduate dentist has had some experience in monetary management, he must hire or train someone to do this for him.

The best way to learn practice management is to work in a dental office as an associate dentist. There you can observe and emulate what successful management looks like. Then, you move on to build or revise your own type of practice management or stay and take over the practice upon retirement of the senior dentist.

After two years of my naval dental service, I returned home and was associated with my family dentist for one year. That was long enough to learn how to manage my own dental practice.

An important lesson from my senior dentist was that our services were fully appreciated only after payment was made in full. Not being a product, dental care service carries a different value concept than things you can buy online or at a shop. This is particularly true when making and delivering removable partial or full dentures. These multiple tooth replacements require time for the patient to learn how to chew comfortably, which is different from treatment of natural teeth. When the appliance is completely paid for and the patient has complete ownership, they always seem to fit and feel better and are accepted by the patient with gratitude.

What kind of dental practice do today's graduates want? Some graduates do not want to manage their own dental practices. They just want to do the dental treatment and leave the management to a manager or some kind of business-management firm. This shift in attitude of recent graduates has occurred for several reasons. Today's graduates face a significant financial burden rather than it being a cultural shift.

The average dental graduate has an onerous school-loan debt of $300,000 to $600,000 that will require many years to repay. They cannot get an additional loan to open their own private practice office. The banks cannot take the risk of loaning even more money to a neophyte, unproven dentist. But more than the large debt that prevents starting a private dental practice is the need to practice new skills of doing general dental treatment. The corporate dental practices have job openings available to attract new dentists wanting this exposure, even though there are significant drawbacks.

What are the drawbacks of choosing to do corporate dentistry? The first one that I know must happen is the scheduling of a high patient volume to maximize profits. The new dentists might have limited time, which could affect the quality of care. After all, after an examination and diagnosis, everything a dentist does is surgical. Most dentists will agree that it takes between five to seven years to be good and fast.

Secondly, corporate dentists work without control over the treatment plans, materials, or the laboratories used. The corporate policies and lay managers can override the dentist's clinical judgment. Thirdly, the treatment options may be limited due to prioritizing production quotas for certain procedures that are more profitable.

Lastly, the lack of clinical autonomy and strict corporate policies based on production over patient care are some of the major drawbacks for dentists opting for corporate practice. My concern is that these for-profit business entities may use the umbrella of the profession to place business interests ahead of patient interests. Until a corporation does something illegal, it is not punished or fined. And until a patient files a complaint about a dentist to the state dental board, there is no investigation. The attorney general of the state or the investigators of the dental board cannot inspect or examine either of these two entities without some complaint by a person who has been injured or cheated. By the time the state dental board or the state corporations have notice to investigate, damage or injury has been done.

Now that the face of dentistry is changing with almost as many women becoming dentists as men, some women dentists choose to take a corporate job, which comes with a dependable salary. This stable option can be appealing to people who juggle most of their family's responsibilities, and it is still the case that our society is more demanding of women than men when it comes to family and household management.

My observations on how long these employees remain with a corporation are purely anecdotal. I have talked to few graduates who have worked for dental corporations. Many of these dentists who start working in corporate practice typically appear to leave after one or two years. Some dentists transition from corporate practice to start their own private practice, join group practices, or find a private practice in which they can build equity and that they can seek to eventually purchase.

The more enterprising young dentists find that corporate employment is not professionally challenging. These clinics address the basic treatment needs of the patients, such as extractions, cleanings, and fillings; but the patients must pay out of pocket for replacement of teeth that are missing. So, they are not as likely to want these services. Prosthetic treatment of tooth replacement for patients is what most general dentists find challenging and gratifying to do. So, they move on to become self-employed in private practice settings. As a private dentist, you can create your own office policies. This will attract patients who want personal dental care, which is more profitable as well.

I believe that if the more savvy or sophisticated young dentists find the boundaries of corporate dentistry too limiting, their patients who are looking for more than just cleanings and fillings will feel the same way.

Because I don't have personal experience with corporate dentistry, aside from the feedback of former dental students, I was driven to do some research about what goes on in these profit motivated practices of dental care because I've heard horror stories.

Back in January 2017, I discovered the settlement of a lawsuit filed by the Texas Attorney General Paxton against MB2 Dental for $8.45 million dollars. Three lawsuits were resolved with this settlement alleging that MB2 knowingly submitted claims for children's dental services that were either not performed or were provided after false identification was used. The claims also involved illegal kickbacks to Medicare and Medicaid beneficiaries and their families, marketers, and marketing entities. The allegations were brought to the attention of the United States and Texas authorities by whistleblowers. The settlement funds will be divided between the whistleblowers, the US government, and the State of Texas.

What was strange was that the MB2 corporation stated the salaried dentists did not do anything wrong. It was probably because they did not even have an inkling of an idea that all this fraudulent activity was going on. The dentists were not held liable for the settlement. The dentists did not have any dealings with the dental services' administration, which is what was fraudulent. This case shows the absolute detachment of the dental providers from the fraudulent billing, phony identification, and kickbacks of three other entities. Although licensed dentists are subject to the regulations and enforcement from the state dental boards, they do not have any say or overview of the financial management or marketing of the corporate entity that they work for.

Another strange aspect of this lawsuit was the fact that MB2 did not admit any guilt. I asked an attorney friend why they did not admit guilt but paid the fine. He told me that these cases are often settled out of court in that manner. No admission of guilt.

I do not mention this lawsuit to infer that all corporate dental practices try to cheat the states and US government for Medicaid programs and their patients. But it does give pause when there are third-party payers, corporate businesspeople, involved with managing large sums of money for health care rather than doctors.

Physicians and dentists manage Health Maintenance Organizations (HMOs). This is where about 24 percent of young dentists are employed to do treatment for Medicaid patients. They must comply with government requirements and are subject to periodic review. So far, there are no separate reviews of these dental corporations by the state dental boards. Time will tell if corporate dentistry can continue to operate in the patient's interest without more reporting to the respective state dental boards.

In the next chapter I'll discuss how the United States government supports health care professions to encourage research and access to health care for the public.

8

COMPETITION FOR HEALTH CARE DOLLAR

The average patient isn't aware of this, but there is a long history of separating dental care from medical care, as if the mouth and the teeth are not related to the care involved for the rest of the body.

To understand the reasons why Medicare does not presently include dental care along with medical care for our senior population, one must know about the historical fragmentation of dentistry from medicine. I have been teaching an elective course on dental history for about ten years as it is no longer a part of the school's required curriculum. This chapter is part of my lecture in the history course to explain how dentistry started out as the poor cousin of medicine. I want my students to understand why their profession was not as highly regarded as the medical field. The reasons behind the exclusion of dental history from educational curriculums remain unclear to me. The curriculum committee in their wisdom obviously felt that it was not that important. I vehemently disagree.

When I was a student, we had a 10-hour course on dental history. I believe before you decide where you want to go, you ought to know where you came from. But I have had to condense the course into two 1-hour sessions. Moreover, I wanted my students to know and be proud of dentistry's contributions to medical surgery. For instance, dentists first discovered and used general anesthesia for painless surgery. This advancement of pre-surgical procedures allowed for longer and more complicated procedures without loss of life.

Dr. Horace Wells was an American dentist who pioneered the use of anesthesia in dentistry and medicine, specifically using nitrous oxide (called laughing gas). This procedure was subsequently adopted by medical surgeons globally. The use of nitrous oxide extended the time available for life-saving procedures. Before it was available for use in surgery, medical operations were of limited time because the patient had to undergo painful surgery and sometimes died of shock if the surgery's duration was too long.

Another major surgical invention by dentistry was

the aspiration (suction) of the bleeding site while doing surgery, so surgeons could better see what they were doing. Up until that time, a surgical nurse had to blot up the obstructing blood with gauze sponges during surgical procedures.. These two inventions became routine in surgery, and revolutionized dental and medical practice.

In the 1800s in the United States, proprietary medical schools trained both medical and dental students together. This method has been used in Europe and is still practiced in some countries today. In several European countries, medical and dental students still train together for the first two years. However, in early America, the dental curriculum part was only one year long. It typically took the last year of a four-year program for dentistry. Prior to the establishment of medical schools that included a dental curriculum, dental practitioners trained by preceptorship. This is where a young person helps an experienced practitioner and watches how treatment procedures are done and assists the senior practitioner. After a few years, the senior practitioner supervises the younger dentist in simpler procedures.

These experienced practitioners also had formed local dental societies among themselves in major American cities and had already produced dental journals for helping fellow practitioners to further educate themselves. They were self-educated by studying the English translation of a book by the French dental surgeon, Dr. Pierre Fauchard. He is called the "Father of Modern Dentistry." In the late 1870s, Dr. Fauchard laid down all the principles of dentistry and described all its various branches within the practice of dentistry, such as orthodontics, oral surgery, prosthetic, restorative, etc. He was an amazing and gifted person who guided American dentists in treatment and knowledge that the medical school deans were not aware of.

As these dental practitioners learned of new treatment procedures, they wanted these procedures to be included in the medical school curriculum for dentists. When dental graduate specialists, known as dentists, approached the medical school dean, they requested an extension of the dental curriculum due to increased knowledge and advancements in dental science. He refused. So, they went off and started the first dental school in the world. The first dental school, the Baltimore College of Dental Surgery, was founded in 1840.

The separation of dental schools from medical schools was influenced by other factors beyond this single reason. The one year dental curriculum was too short to include all the new knowledge from lectures by prominent dentists to medical and dental students. Dentists requested the inclusion of their expertise in the curriculum, but this proposal was not adopted by the medical school administration.

Later, dentists in other states started other dental schools in the US for similar reasons. Dental schools became competitive institutions that attracted potential medical students who wanted to become dental specialists (dentists), away from the medical schools.

This schism became wider as time went on and resulted in a loss of income for medical school owners. Worse yet, these disgruntled owners looked down on the startup dental schools and claimed the dental students there were not as well trained. They said that these dentists did not graduate from a medical school where they teach about the rest of the body. The dental school deans responded to these accusations by saying that their dental students received four years of training, of which the latter two years were with dental clinical training that medical schools did not provide.

There may have been partial truth in these accusations of not having enough knowledge of the rest of the body. Medical school deans were critical of the dental schools during the late 1800s. Strangely enough, medical practice laws and regulations allow the physician to treat the entire body, mouth and teeth included, even though they are not trained in the anatomy, diagnosis, or treatment of the teeth and gums. Dentistry should be recognized as a branch of medicine. As dentists became more knowledgeable about the rest of the body and their dental skills, as well, the public perception of dentistry as a separate profession was shifting.

I believe that a lesser factor leading to a subordinate role of dentists to physicians may be due to the accepted contraction of two words, dental specialist, to dentist. We were not called dental doctors or mouth doctors. Then when people referred to health care providers, they started calling us, collectively, doctors and dentists. As if dentists were not deserving of the name doctor. Or implying that dental services were not as critical to one's health as other forms of medical treatment. Graduates of dental schools are generally given a degree of Doctor of Dental Surgery (DDS). Certain dental schools, however, confer the degree of Doctor of Dental Medicine (DMD).

Throughout history, dental surgeons (dentists) performed oral surgeries while physicians avoided surgery until the Renaissance allowed anatomical dissection. The reason some dental schools started to give Doctor of Dental Medicine degrees was to emphasize that dental services were medically based as well. In the early 1900s, combined medical and dental schools were known as Colleges of Physicians and Surgeons, with dentists referred to as surgeons. My school (UOP) was formerly called by this name, and one dental school, at Columbia University in New York City, still retains the name of College of Physicians and Surgeons.

The training of most medical students does not include anything about dental health. They may have a visiting dental professor lecture once or twice about the importance of dental health. While my son was attending Tulane University's medical school, it was recommended that he study a book on oral pathology to gain comprehensive knowledge about diseases of the mouth. The students there were told to refer a patient to a dentist if that patient had pain or discomfort in the head or mouth that the doctor could not diagnose. Since the medical students never learned about dental health, they assumed that the health of teeth and mouth were not important to one's general health. What is even stranger is that most state medical licenses allow physicians to treat any part of the body. In fact, it was not until 1999 that the Surgeon General of the United States declared that you cannot have good general health without good dental health. Medical doctors now understand that oral health affects overall health.

The schism between the two professions became wider as the US government began more health care programs. Health care for the merchant mariners during post-colonial times was one of the first areas of government intervention of health services of this essential occupation. The country depended on goods both exported and imported by sea for a stable and growing economy. Subsequently, the US Public Health Service was founded to provide health services to these mariners. All the appropriation bills of Congress depended on lobbying funds during the 1900s. Later on, prior to WWII, the medical lobby would tell Congress, the dentists just save teeth; we save lives. This lobbying tactic resulted in the medical lobby getting the lion's share of the health care dollars. This kind of mentality continued among legislators and some of the public until the beginning of World War II in 1941.

During military conscription, or the draft during WWII, the induction of young men into the military services revealed that the main reason for not being physically fit to serve was poor dental health. Able-bodied young men with eight or more missing teeth or a lot of badly decayed teeth, were turned away; they were not turned away for flat feet. The main reason oral health is so important for the soldiers and sailors was their ability to effectively chew their food and not have any toothaches. The so-called "K rations" often contained hard foods that would not easily spoil. I remember after WWII, trying to bite into a surplus K ration chocolate bar that was so hard, I could only break off a piece with a kitchen knife. In addition, a soldier or sailor must be free of toothaches to function effectively.

When the military high command heard about why young able-bodied men were most often rejected, dental health was given the same importance as medical health. Thanks to military experience, both medical and dental services were recognized as being equally important for maintaining the health of the armed forces. This resulted in the parity of salaries between medical and dental officers. Interestingly, the dental officers in the US Army and US Air Force are under the command of their respective medical corps.

The navy had learned the importance of dental health earlier. Sailors on ships are far from land-based dental clinics. The Navy Dental Corp was established in 1912 and has its own high-ranking dental admirals, separate from the army and air force medical corps.

Like flight surgeons (medical doctors) who were attached to naval squadrons, I was also attached to a squadron as a flight dental officer. In the early 1960s, when I was a young navy dental officer, at one of two major training centers in San Diego, California, some of our recruits from poor areas of the country had to be separated out and placed in a "dental company." This allowed a longer training period due to the extensive need for more dental appointments for missing or decayed teeth that had to be treated. There were very few ships that had dentists onboard to take care of dental problems. At that time, only carriers, cruisers, and supply ships had a dentist and dental clinics onboard.

Furthermore, the Navy Dental Corp has recognized the education and the ability of its dental officers in the surgical operating rooms aboard ships and onshore during wartime. The duties of the dental officers include assisting the medical surgeons with general anesthesia during combat because more anesthesiologists are needed than are available. Dental officers attached to the marines are also trained to direct the navy medical corpsman in triage procedures to identify the condition of the wounded and recognize fatal injuries on the battlefield. Also, in wartime the dentist operates the morgue because dentists are uniquely qualified to identify the mortally wounded sailors and marines by inspection of dental records.

While the military does offer dental services, there are still strict standards on oral health to prevent the need for excessive dental treatment during active duty. Imagine all the liabilities that can happen with a toothache or infection and the inability to eat properly. Regular checkup visits to the dental clinic are encouraged and mandatory when on active duty. I know that our navy flying personnel were assigned flight dentists, such as myself, to ensure everyone on flight status had periodic preventive dental care. I believe that the government's experience with military health care led to the recognition that it was not possible to have good general health without good dental health. The military command of the armed forces clearly acknowledges the equal importance of both dental and medical care for the health and wellbeing of soldiers, sailors, marines, and pilots.

Despite dentistry's recognition by the military, medical care receives the lion's share of health care dollars because of the larger amount of medical research. The main causes for death are related to cardiovascular diseases, cancer, and respiratory diseases. Medicine was first in line to get funding for medical research that might lead to increased longevity. In the early 1950s, research in dentistry was still ongoing, but dental issues rarely advanced to early death because a tooth extraction could avoid serious consequences. By this time, medicine had soaked up most of the research funding. Finally, after establishing our own National Institute of Dental and Craniofacial Research (NIDCR) under the National Institutes of Health (NIH) in 1998, we began to receive more research dollars—especially when the research began on the gums or gingival tissues with the use of the electron microscope. Crossover diseases, such as cardiovascular disease and the low birth weight of infants, have now encouraged joint research by the two professions. Healthy teeth and gums are crucial for the effective treatment of medical diseases.

Another reason dentistry wasn't included in Medicare is that, in the 1960s and 1970s, most dentists didn't want to participate in government health programs. They were wary that the government would limit the patient to the less costly, temporary kinds of treatment.

Under California's Denti-Cal program, which is partially federally funded, dentists were initially limited to performing root canal treatments only on front teeth, not back teeth. Back teeth have more root canals and are more costly to treat. But back teeth are necessary for chewing food. Chewing with the front teeth alone will loosen the teeth under the muscular strain placed on them. Finally, after suing the state program, we prevailed and could then thoroughly treat patients and save the more costly back teeth too.

Medical care coverage, be it as Medicare, Medicaid, or Denti Cal, often places restrictions on the services dentists can provide. But we dentists can solve the problem of replacing missing teeth four or five separate ways. We did not want to rely on the government's choice for replacing missing teeth. For this reason, the ADA did not try to lobby Congress to be included in government programs. We knew from the state programs for the indigent, that the government would choose the cheapest way to solve the tooth-loss problem. This may not necessarily be in the interest of the patient but determined by the penny-pinching of the government.

The dentists in California were encouraged by our professional organization, the California Dental Association (CDA), to take care of at least a few Denti-Cal or Medicaid patients. So, I did. At the time, several years ago, I was paying the going salary rate of fifty dollars per patient to my dental hygienist for her services. She would usually see one patient per hour. I had about five patients in my private dental practice that applied for and received Medicaid Denti-Cal benefits. I recommended the patients see me semiannually for an examination by me and teeth cleaning by my hygienist. But the state program only allowed this procedure once a year and paid me twenty-five dollars per patient. Well, how long can you conduct the business part of your dental practice that way? I decided to find the time to take care of these patients myself because I wasn't going to pay my hygienist twice the amount of money that I received from the state. This is the experience we have with state government programs, and it hasn't gotten much better from what I hear.

Today, many of the younger dentists are more willing to go along with Medicare reimbursement, as long as the overhead costs are considered. I say that because our overhead is barely covered by present-day state and federal funding; that funding is below our costs for Denti-Cal programs in

California. In the reimbursement for surgical medical care, the medical surgeons are always paid more than some of the other physicians. However, all general dentists are surgeons. We have to pay for our office expenses, unlike the medical surgeons who just go to a hospital to treat the patient without the high overhead that the dentist has in his private setting.

Almost every procedure the dentist does is surgical, e.g. cutting hard and soft tissue, such as, teeth and bone, or the soft tissues of the gums. When not performing surgical treatments, dentists provide services that can involve prosthetic care, which includes paying a dental laboratory to make a crown, bridgework, or a denture.

Most dentists have an overhead expense of 75 to 80 percent compared to medical doctor office visits of 35 to 40 percent overhead. What our government likes to ignore is that the overhead cost of dental practice is about two times (or greater) compared to that of medical practice. All private dental practices have equipment costs, such as X-ray machines, dental chairs, hand instrument costs, laboratory costs, sterilization costs, local anesthetic and dental anesthesia costs, and restorative material costs. We are doing hard and soft tissue surgery in a hospital-like setting. We make prosthetic appliances and restorations of teeth that require precision accuracy within tenths of one millimeter, and we have laboratory bills to pay. All of this care can be done without going to the hospital. This is why dental office care costs more than medical office care but is far less expensive than hospital care.

With the increased presence of dental assistants and dental hygienists, a general dentist can care for many more patients than in the years past. Also, there are now several more dental schools in the country graduating more dentists than before. Fifty years ago, there were about fifty dental schools in the US. Now there are seventy-two dental schools here, and Canada has ten dental schools. The demographics for the ratio of dentists to patients has changed, so younger dentists are not as busy and are more willing to treat patients who are on government-subsidized dental care programs, such as Medicaid and Medicare. Presently, and for the last few years, the ADA has lobbied Congress for inclusion of dental services for Medicare patients.

In the near future, it is anticipated that Medicare will offer limited dental services. Similar to how drug costs are currently managed separately, these services will likely be included as an optional choice for patients. But the allowable fees must be usual, customary, and reasonable (UCR). Otherwise, most dentists will not participate in these government programs.

Moreover, there are now attempts by medical and dental schools to bring the professions of dentistry and medicine closer together for the improvement of treatment that involve diseases of the mouth or gums and other organs of the body. Here in California, my dental school (UOP) has been funded to join a medical school in the Sacramento area to train medical and dental residents under the same roof. A medical school has yet to be chosen for this program. The students will have joint courses and learn about each other's profession. They will be able to discuss a patient's disease, such as diabetes, face to face across disciplines.

While dentistry and medicine needed separation 170 years ago to advance dental sciences, they now must collaborate in research of diseases affecting multiple body areas. For instance, diabetes is a perfect example of a systemic disease that has a two-way relationship with gum disease. The people with diabetes are more likely to have gum problems, and gum problems can lead to worsening of the control of diabetes. This systemic disease has a two-way relationship between metabolic and periodontal disease. You cannot have one without the other.

At a continuing-education lecture I attended recently, I heard about a joint medical research project between a physician researcher at Stanford Medical School and one of our oral surgeon researchers at the UOP Dugoni School of Dentistry. This collaborative research on crossover diseases will justify the historical linkages between dentistry and medicine, for example, if the research shows direct causation of gingivitis or periodontitis with a more serious systemic disease.

Even though dentistry is the largest branch of medicine, our profession does not receive anywhere near the research funds that go to address cancer, cardiovascular, and respiratory diseases. Of the 48 billion dollars of fund spent in 2020 for medical research, dentistry's budget portion was 404 million dollars. In other words, less than one percent of research funding money.

Of course, these areas of medicine can result in life-threatening maladies, called comorbidities. Early diagnosis and treatment of heart, lung and prostrate diseases are the main reasons for prolonging longevity or increasing the lifespan of our people. But public health measures seen on TV, such as encouraging people to avoid smoking and labeling alcoholic beverages to limit drinking, are making a difference to prevent these primary illnesses. I would like to see the CDC and the ADA do more public health information campaigns on the importance of dental checkup visits to prevent both dental and medical diseases. Once dental care becomes available to Medicare folks, the need for dental care will be comparable to the need for medical care.

Government programs do not cover cosmetic dentistry, which will be discussed in the next chapter.

9

COSMETIC DENTISTRY

Poets and writers have waxed eloquent about the beauty of a smile for centuries. Of how our teeth are like dancing pearls on a stage of lips. Are our teeth not part of the beauty of a smile? Just try to smile without showing your teeth. Your smile will appear forced or phony. When teeth show, it is so much more genuine a smile. It is romantic but true: a returned smile from across the room can lead to the beginning of a relationship.

The American public puts a great deal of value on the way their teeth look. This is truer here than any other people I have seen when traveling outside the country. This observation becomes evident when you see how people want to have bathtub-white teeth. Now, they can whiten them themselves, without going to the dentist.

I can understand why celebrities and TV newscasters want their teeth to be very white. It is because they are in a studio under artificial lighting or in the public spotlight.

However, most other people overdo the bleaching of their teeth. When used properly, cosmetics and hair coloring products can enhance a person's appearance in a way that looks natural and youthful. Artfully done, cosmetics make us look and feel better. Tooth bleaching can be done to make darkened teeth look lighter and natural if it is done artfully.

Moreover, if a patient bleaches their teeth too long with a powerful bleaching agent, it can cause tooth sensitivity to cold water, iced drinks, or some acidic foods like vinegar. I have had to help patients with these problems of over bleaching by prescribing desensitizing toothpastes.

There are multiple foods, drinks, and habits that can stain your teeth. Even though the enamel of a tooth is the hardest biological tissue in our body, it is porous to some degree. This allows the enamel of teeth to absorb the color of things we drink and eat, such as coffee, teas, wine, beets, blueberries, and blackberries. Our teeth can be stained by a tobacco habit as well, and not just on the surface;

teeth can become tobacco-stained from deep within the dentin.

When I had patients who wanted me to bleach their teeth, before all these bleaching products were available to the public, I told them that I would help them, but I wanted them to understand that the perceived degree of whiteness of their teeth was related to their complexion, which needed to be considered to not overdo bleaching. In other words, if they had a dark skin tone, their tooth color would always look lighter by comparison. In fact, people of color have darker teeth, however, their teeth look like they are whiter than people with lighter skin tones because of the contrasting difference.

Everyone wants whiter and more beautiful teeth. Now that it is safe to purchase tooth-bleaching products and do it yourself, too many people are over-bleaching their teeth. Teeth can appear to look bathtub white and artificially fake to me. Moreover, you do not have to be a dentist to spot artificially whitened teeth.

Therefore, my advice is not to overdo tooth bleaching. Your teeth may become stained by tea, coffee, smoking, or drinking red wine. If you want to have lighter-looking teeth, it is a clever idea to first have your teeth cleaned professionally to remove any stains that may be on the surface.

Then, if you still feel they are not as light as before, try tooth bleaching. Ask your dentist to guide you to a shade that is lighter but still looks natural. This would require a short return visit that your dentist would not even charge you for. But ask, in advance. In this way, you would have your dentist's professional judgment as to what degree of lightness is attractive and natural.

Fortunately, teeth can be whitened or bleached safely for people over the age of twenty-one. I don't recommend teenagers bleach their teeth because the nerve (dental pulp) is still large. Their teeth are more sensitive to the powerful effects of the bleaching process. As we become older, the nerve size diminishes, and the teeth become less sensitive.

The best way to improve the alignment for better esthetics is by moving the natural teeth by orthodontic treatment. Yes, it takes longer, and it is more expensive. However, your tooth retains the layer of enamel that protects it from dental decay. The tooth is also stronger and can resist fracture when you save as much enamel as possible. This a good reason not to have veneers which requires enamel reduction to look natural.

Traditional orthodontics and plastic aligners technique are the most lasting solutions for tooth-alignment issues. The use of multiple dental splint retainers—Invisalign is the most common brand used—to realign your front teeth depends on Computer Aided Design and Computer Aided Manufacturing (CAD-CAM), a computer-driven technology. This treatment can correct about 25 percent of malocclusion (crooked front teeth). This treatment is very popular but cannot be used successfully when a more serious malocclusion is present.

I can tell you that so much cosmetic dentistry has depended upon technological advances from research to producing revolutionary changes in our dental materials. For instance, the most common choice used for filling and restoring teeth are bonded composites. They not only can match the shade of a tooth almost perfectly but can be done in one appointment. After multiple generations and successive reiterations over the last sixty years, composite bonding materials can bond to the tooth enamel and not require tooth cutting down to hold the filling material. In years past, fillings had to be held by tooth reduction. Moreover, this treatment is the least costly.

The bonding of composite materials is used for restoring decayed teeth as well as augmentation of a chipped, broken, or misaligned tooth. Composites are the most widely used dental material and have reduced the need to provide a crown in many cases. Also, composites cost much less than crowns and they can be done in one visit, which also leads to cost reduction.

Sometimes using the bonding of a composite to your tooth, as mentioned, can improve the aesthetics, such as in the case of a fractured tooth. I was trained to conserve the enamel and find ways to remove as little as possible when solving an aesthetic or restorative problem. Bonding is a better procedure than veneers because it does not remove a lot of enamel like veneers do. After all, enamel is the hardest biological tissue in animals and the human dentition. But it does not grow back and repair itself like many of our other tissues.

An artificial crown covers the whole tooth by reducing all enamel and some dentin to allow for a jacket-like cover. This procedure duplicates all the anatomy of the original natural crown. However, most composite bonding cannot last as long as a crown. I always like to explain to a patient when a choice or option is available. After all, a composite may have to be replaced due to wear or fracture. Still the cost difference is often worth trying the less costly procedure first. On the other hand, consider paying more for the most natural and long-lasting result. The takeaway recommendation is to always ask your dentist for alternative treatment choices.

Porcelain laminates or porcelain and composite veneers are another cosmetic option. Porcelain and composite veneers can be cemented to your teeth that are not straight, or even used to avoid needing orthodontic treatment that takes a lot longer to accomplish. While composite veneers are cheaper, I recommend porcelain veneers for their stain resistance and natural appearance. The patient who wants this kind of cosmetic treatment should be willing to have the most natural and long-lasting result. Besides, composite veneers do not have the luster of porcelain.

Now that you know all about the ins and outs of porcelain veneers, I must tell you I do not recommend them most of the time to improve the looks of your teeth. There are two or three other ways to solve your needs that I believe are better solutions.

Porcelain veneers can be done to improve the looks or alignment of your teeth. However, almost all the enamel on the front of your teeth must be shaved off to allow space for the veneer. Once this procedure has been done, it may have to be redone, some years later. After a period of ten to twenty years, your gums usually will recede to the point of exposing the edge of the veneer. If you have a high lip-line smile, you may want to have the veneers redone to look more natural.

Full-crown coverage is yet another longer-lasting way to achieve better aesthetics and strength. The porcelains used today have been vacuum-fired and hardened to resist fracture almost as well as metal does. For even greater strength in a crown treatment, porcelain can be fused to the underlying metal of a crown.. Ideally, the metal used is a white-gold alloy, not a non-precious metal, which is cheaper. A non-precious metal is much more difficult to work with for adjustment of the newly made restoration to the opposing chewing tooth surfaces.

The marginal fit is better with using precious metal than non-precious because the alloy containing gold is more malleable. I recommend and used these porcelain-fused-to-white-gold crowns more frequently; because they can have the porcelain on the lip or cheek side that shows and a white-gold on the chewing surface. This design is best as the gold is softer than the non-precious metal and can provide the same rate of wear as the opposing teeth's natural enamel. This type of crown has the aesthetics of porcelain to match the shade of the adjacent teeth, and the lasting wearability of white-gold.

All-porcelain crowns are frequently advised for comprehensive coverage of a fractured tooth or to reinforce a weakened tooth. But this material can be very abrasive and can cause undue wear on the opposing natural teeth. When given the option, ask your dentist for the white-gold alloy fused to porcelain crown if you want the most lasting and aesthetic treatment. It can be used on front teeth as well, although the aesthetics of all-porcelain are better on front teeth, all-porcelain is not as strong.

When a tooth is missing and needs replacement, the ideal choice is a tooth implant. I would typically offer my patient the choice of bridgework or implants. Bridgework requires the placement of a crown on either side of the missing tooth or teeth to hold the pontic (dummy tooth) replacement. The bridgework is attached permanently by cementation to the nearby teeth. Implants involve a different process. The implant body is surgically placed in the jawbone, and a crown is placed upon it. Both types of treatment, bridgework or implant, can be suitable to restore a natural look cosmetically. But implants can simulate the natural function of missing teeth as well as the beauty of natural teeth.

There are two main categories of dental prostheses for replacing missing teeth. One is removable prosthesis like partial dentures or full dentures. The other is fixed prosthesis using bridgework or bone-supported implants. Fixed bridgework, which must be cemented to adjacent supporting teeth, was the only popular option for many years. Bridgework is still useful and costs less than implants. Bridgework requires cleaning under dummy teeth daily or after dinner. An implant is like having a natural tooth. Brushing and flossing it is like cleaning your natural teeth. Dentists only dreamed of implant dentistry sixty years ago. Implants do cost more than bridgework because of the surgical procedure to place the implant body into the jawbone.

Bridgework has limitations because it relies on support from adjacent teeth which must be carry the load of the missing teeth. If too many teeth need to be replaced, then a removable partial denture can be designed. This option is always better than complete full-denture replacement. Well-designed partial dentures can be tooth-plus-jawbone supported for comfortable chewing and esthetics. However, they must be cleaned after meals as food particles can accumulate under the prosthesis.

All general dentists are trained to do cosmetic dentistry. (Although some dentists limit their practices to concentrating on cosmetics.) When restoring teeth, the aesthetics of the teeth is an important consideration. Dentists are trained to match the shade of filling material or crowns to the adjacent natural teeth. We can, for instance, prepare before-and-after models to show our patients what enhancements can be done with one method or another, before deciding on what looks best.

Fortunately, there are now software programs that can create what your teeth can look like using different treatment modalities. These software programs save a lot of time and laboratory work. It can give the patient a more lifelike look at what is obtainable in enhancement before going ahead with treatment. So, as you can see, dental training is not limited to the dental sciences alone; dentists are trained to be artistic as well.

Much of my training in facial artistry came from being trained to restore a patient's natural facial features when replacing all of their teeth with full dentures. As students, we not only learned the anatomy of the various bony structures of the jaws to build the false teeth onto, but we had to learn the anatomical structures of the face as well. After all, our teeth and supporting bones support our lips and cheeks.

As an aside, by the time of his inauguration, our first president, George Washington, had lost all but one of his teeth. When he was asked to sit for the artist to do a portrait for the engraving for the one-dollar bill, the artist demanded to confer with the president's dentist, Dr. John Greenwood. Washington's false teeth left his mouth looking caved in and unnatural. The artist asked Dr. Greenwood to make special appliances for Washington to wear during the artist sitting, so Washington's face would look natural. Dr. Greenwood designed upper and lower dentures made from lead, which the president only wore during the artistic seatings. So, President Washington looked better on the one-dollar bill than he did in real life.

When restoring front teeth with crowns, bridgework, or implants, I asked patients to bring their spouse or significant other to the final appointment. I requested this because I wanted a family member or friend beside the patient, to approve the aesthetics of my work. After all, it is your family and friends who must look at your teeth and appearance. I did not want my patient to go home and have an important person in their life not approve of the result.

Another way that I showed my patient what a treatment would look like was a trial placement of front-teeth restorations. I required my patient to get out of the chair and come to a wall mirror to first view what the new treatment was to look like. I would have them stand at a conversational distance to view their teeth first. Then I would ask them for their approval before I let them get closer. The reason I asked them to be stepped-back from the mirror is that it is next to impossible to perfectly duplicate a natural tooth sitting next to an artificial one. I knew some older dentists who would not replace or crown a single front central tooth; they would insist on doing additional preparation of yet another healthy tooth, so the front two teeth would match. But I chose to have my patients understand the limitations of my care.

Because I used a dental laboratory that was nearby, I would often have my assigned dental technician come to my office and do a shade match of my patient's teeth. I did not want to rely on a picture or my judgment alone. In this way, my patient knew that I did everything possible to achieve the best shade match of their adjacent teeth. My lab man could also vary from the standard shades with special tinting to match the patient's tooth shade.

Your smile depends a great deal upon the appearance and beauty of your dentition. But the health of your mouth and the structures within are, of course, more important than the way your teeth look. Imagine trying to speak, sing, or eat without your natural teeth. Without a mouthful of healthy teeth and gums, the pleasures of living would be sorely compromised. Although cosmetic dentistry has encouraged patients to seek dental treatment, the attending dentist must always place the health of your mouth above the wants or needs for beautiful teeth. The smart and dentally sophisticated patient should rely on their general dentist's opinion of cosmetic enhancement of teeth before trying to find a so-called cosmetic dentist. A dentist with a practice limited to "cosmetic dentistry"—which is not a recognized specialty by the ADA—may overlook making certain that no disease conditions exist before starting cosmetic treatment.

However, I have on a few occasions referred my patient to a local dentist who was known to do cosmetic dentistry. I felt they could do better than I could do. Or, I referred out if I felt I could not meet my patient's expectations. Of course, I could assure my patient that their mouth was free of any dental disease before sending them to someone for cosmetic treatment. Furthermore, I would not recommend going to a dentist who only advertises cosmetic dentistry services. Stating this claim on TV or in a newspaper does not make one any better at what they can do. Obtaining a referral from your dentist gives you confidence that the referred dentist does really provide superior cosmetic treatment.

There are numerous options available to enhance dental aesthetics and achieve an improved smile. Take the time to discuss with your general dentist the various ways you can achieve the look you want. You have a trusted relationship with your dentist for the maintenance of better dental health. And your dentist may be able to do the cosmetic treatment to your satisfaction or recommend someone who can better address your needs. Very few dentists specialize in cosmetic dentistry. Cosmetic dentistry is widely practiced but not an ADA-recognized specialty.

In the next chapter I will talk about what the dental specialty services focus on.

10

DENTAL SPECIALTIES

Most often a general practitioner of dentistry attends patients because they are trained in all aspects of dentistry. However, when treatment is more complicated or the general dentist feels that a specialist can better serve the patient, the patient may be referred to one of thirteen specialists: An Orthodontist; Oral/maxillofacial surgeon; Periodontist; Pediatric dentist; Endodontist; Prosthodontist; Orthodontist; Dental radiologist; Oral pathologist; Dental anesthesiologist; Oral medicine specialist; Orofacial pain specialist; and a Public health dentist.

The general dentist is responsible for your long-term dental care, whereas the specialists are interested in the limited care of their specialty. Although a patient may go directly to a specialist for treatment, insurance companies often make consultation with a general dentist necessary before any treatment by a specialist.

The most common reason to seek a specialist is when parents want to have orthodontic treatment to straighten their child's teeth. They may consult their general dentist whom they have had a long relationship with for a referral to an orthodontist. Or they may wish to choose an orthodontist whom they have been referred to by another parent. After an initial examination by the orthodontist, the orthodontist may decide to recommend the removal of the child's four wisdom (third molar) teeth or removal of two or four second bicuspid teeth. At this point, the parents may just go along with this decision or seek more advice. This is when going back to your general dentist for, yet another opinion is very helpful.

If both the orthodontist and the general practitioner agree that certain teeth should be removed for effective orthodontic treatment, a referral to an oral surgeon may be needed. Your general dentist may feel that an oral surgeon can best perform wisdom teeth (third molar) extractions. However, the general practitioner may say that they can extract the bicuspids, since they are confident in their ability to extract these teeth.

Some general dentists can implement nitrous oxide gas sedation or twilight sleep to their patient by intravenous injection or by oral medication. But most dentists are not trained as well as oral surgeons to administer different levels of anesthesia.

Now, if all these teeth need to be extracted, both wisdom and bicuspid teeth before beginning the orthodontic treatment, it may be in the best interest of the child to have an oral surgeon do all of the molar extractions in one appointment. It would not be advisable to schedule two surgical appointments when all the treatment could be done in just one appointment. Or the bicuspid teeth could all be removed at one appointment. Consultation with your family dentist can be an invaluable help in making these decisions.

Let's look at each specialty, one by one, as these specialties represent the experts in the dental field.

Oral/maxillofacial surgeon

Oral surgeons are frequently required to perform complex tooth extractions or conduct soft tissue biopsies on suspicious lesions. Most oral surgeons have hospital privileges and can administer general anesthesia (GA) in their office as well.

In treatment of an implanted tooth, oral surgeons and periodontists are also the best specialists to provide the insertion of implant body for the patient. Then the general dentist or prosthodontist can place or cement a crown on the implant to complete the tooth replacement. The implant body is the infrastructure of an implanted tooth that the oral surgeon places in the jawbone. Then the general dentist or prosthodontist places the crown or constructs a bridge upon the implant body.

I would often refer my younger patients to an oral surgeon when they needed to have one or more of their third molar teeth (wisdom) removed if the teeth were impacted or unable to erupt from the jawbone into the mouth. These molars erupt when young women are between eighteen and twenty-two, thus they are called wisdom teeth. Young men have the wisdom teeth emerge at twenty-one to twenty-five years of age. Wisdom teeth are the most troublesome of all one's teeth and are sometimes not present, or one or two may be missing. Many times, these teeth are anomalies with odd or weird crown and root shapes.

If a wisdom tooth is causing pain from a gum infection around the tooth, called a pericoronitis flap infection, the removal of the gum tissue or extraction of the tooth may be necessary. Oral surgeons often do this procedure.

Oral surgeons do biopsies of suspicious lesions and

do bone grafts to increase the thickness and bone height for an implant or a removable prosthesis, such as a partial or full denture. Removal of impacted lower wisdom teeth are best done by an oral surgeon due to their expertise in conserving as much surrounding jawbone as possible. What I mean here is that the expertise of tooth extraction is the ability to remove a tooth that is encased in bone, done in a way that minimizes the loss of bone tissue. Oral surgeons are also knowledgeable about the proximity of the mandibular nerve to the roots of these teeth. The use of extraoral panoramic X-rays is necessary to see the exact location of these anatomical structures. As you can see, oral surgeons have expertise and routinely perform complicated surgical procedures.

Periodontist

Periodontists are specialists in gums and gum diseases. They perform gingival (gum) or deep gum curettage and/or surgery of the gums and bone tissues in instances of advanced periodontal disease. They are also well trained in the management and placement of implants. As is often necessary, periodontists can reshape the bone around some of the teeth. The success of periodontal surgery depends on the patient's home care and ability to floss thoroughly before and after the surgery.

Usually, the periodontist will not begin surgical treatment until the patient can learn to properly floss their teeth. The surgery will fail if the patient does not floss regularly, and properly, after the gum surgery. So, periodontists have their staff teach patients proper flossing habits before surgical treatment.

My periodontist used to have a butcher's five-inch hook tied and hanging down from his dental lamp. With it dangling there, it would not take long for a patient to ask what the hook was there for. The periodontist would smile and tell them, "That is where I hang patients who do not floss their teeth." Sometimes a joke helps to instill the importance of doing more than just brushing. Upon completion of the periodontal treatment, the periodontist would normally return the patient back to the referring dentist for continued well-patient care of periodic examinations of the teeth and for oral cancer screening. Most periodontists will also want to examine the patient's gum health annually as a follow-up. In most cases, these patients needed more frequent visits for teeth cleaning and reexamination of the periodontal pocket depths.

Many periodontists can also place the implant body for a patient because periodontists work with reshaping the bone around teeth as well as the gums. They then would refer the patient back to the general dentist or prosthodontist for the final crown restoration.

Pediatric Dentist

The pediatric dentist is a children's dentist. If the general (family) dentist does not treat children or the child needs special management for their care, the general dentist may recommend a pedodontist. Most pediatric dentists are trained to place a child under sedation to render their care, only if necessary. They may use nitrous oxide or intravenous sedation. The pediatric dentist may also do early orthodontic treatment, as they have more advanced training in children's developmental dentition. They will usually refer their teenage patients back to a general dentist when the second molar eruptions are completed, around the age of fourteen to sixteen years of age. The pediatric dental staff should show parents how to floss their child's teeth starting around two and a half years old. This is when the primary premolar teeth have erupted and are touching one another, unlike the separated front teeth of a child. Without proper flossing, these premolars, which remain in the mouth until a child is around thirteen years old, are the earliest teeth to have a cavity.

The reception areas of pediatric dental offices are

arranged to be inviting for families with young children. They often feature toys and coloring pages to keep children engaged while they wait. Moreover, the staff is specially trained so that children have an enjoyable and fun visit and look forward to returning periodically.

Although I did not have toys in my reception area, I took care of my own children and some of their little friends because much of their care was well-patient care. This means it was preventive checkups with very few cavities to treat. However, I must say that I had an extensive course in pediatric care and treated my nephews and nieces, as well as many children, while at dental school. My dental school required two 10-week clinics, one after the second year and another after the third year. At the summer clinics we worked from 8 a.m. to 5 p.m. with no lectures or time off. Most schools did not have summer clinics or just had one. In addition, one of the so-called Fathers of Children's Dentistry, Dr. Charles Sweet, was not only a graduate of my school, but he was also still on the faculty during my training.

Endodontist

The endodontist does root canal treatment (endodontics) to save and maintain a tooth in which the nerve has become abscessed or infected. After removing the nerve and sterilizing the root canal, the canal is filled with an inert substance to preserve the tooth. The endodontist is specially trained to do retreatment of root canal teeth that have become reinfected. The endodontist is also able to provide extra sedation for his patients. Some of the back teeth have two, three or four nerve canals that are more complicated to treat than the front teeth, which usually have only one nerve. Most general dentists are trained to do root canal treatment but prefer to refer the complicated back molars and/or some bicuspid teeth surgeries to an endodontist.

All endodontists have specialized microscopes to do their treatment while using 25-times magnification, which can reveal hidden root canals that are critical to achieving a successful result. This microscope allows the operator to magnify a pinhole speck of a root canal to appear the size of an eraser end of a wooden pencil. Many endodontists also use the cone beam X-ray machine to show hundreds of slices of minute details in three dimensions to better see the exact extent of the root canal. The endodontically treated tooth can now be retained healthfully, providing the surrounding gum tissues are healthy. A crown and/or post might be required to reinforce the tooth. If a significant portion of the coronal structure is absent, a crown or post is recommended as there may be an insufficient amount of the crown left, due to decay or fracture.

Now that implant dentistry is available, there is a question of whether an infected tooth should be treated by endodontic treatment or by the option of the tooth being extracted and replaced with an implant. However, if the nerve of the diseased tooth has healthy gum around it and is immobile and the bone infection is minimal, I would recommend endodontic treatment instead of an implant. Once the diseased nerve is removed, the body will heal the bone infection, and a patient can avoid the more involved surgery and the greater cost of an implant.

Endodontic offices are always ready to accept emergency patients with a painful tooth. Sometimes, the general dentist cannot easily interrupt his treatment to relieve a patient with a painful toothache. But I have never had to call more than one endodontist to help my patient in pain when I could not serve them immediately.

Prosthodontist

The prosthodontist replaces teeth for patients who have more complex needs, such as several missing teeth or no existing teeth. Some general dentists do not treat patients without any teeth because their training was not sufficient for that situation, or they just prefer to treat patients with their own natural teeth. Prosthodontists can make full dentures, or removable partial dentures if enough teeth are present. They can do full-mouth rehabilitation, which requires bridgework, multiple crowns, and/or implants.

My office was in a medical/dental building with over 350 dentists and physicians. Some of the younger dentists in the building referred their full-denture patients to me because they knew I didn't mind taking care of older folks who had no natural teeth.

Over the years I referred many patients to various specialists. One of these patients was the fifth, and last wife, Betty Lin, of the celebrated singer, Eddie Fisher She referred him to me for prosthetic treatment. He was having a difficult time just chewing food as the blade implants in three of the four quadrants of his mouth were coming loose. The blade implant was a type of implant that preceded the present type of implants, and many of Eddie's were unsuccessful and became infected and had to be replaced. Eddie was found by my patient, Betty Lin, a very successful businesswoman, in a drug recovery program in the Haight-Ashbury district of San Francisco. She rescued him medically, dentally, and financially, then helped him restart his professional career. He was grateful for whatever I could do for him, but his dental problems involved major full-mouth rehabilitation. Eddie's restorative problems were greater than my ability to treat, so I referred him to a prosthodontist. He needed to have extractions of all but one of the blade implants, which was done by an oral surgeon, plus bone grafting. Then he had to immediately have temporary removable teeth made that served until the permanent bridgework and implants could be completed. The implants were placed to support a bridge on one side, while the natural teeth supported another bridge on the upper jaw. The lower jaw required a spark erosion bar plus four implants and crowns for a removable partial denture. After more than a year of this extensive dental treatment, the prosthodontist sent him back to me for routine dental care.

Orthodontist

The only specialist treatment Eddie Fisher did not need was orthodontic care. The orthodontist straightens and realigns teeth for children and adults. This treatment usually takes more than one year. Sometimes, orthodontic care is required to expand the palatal bone of the upper arch of the teeth of a child before orthodontic movement of the teeth. They also can do treatment with multiple retainers, like Invisalign, in place of braces, in less complicated conditions. Some parents believe this treatment is purely cosmetic. However, people with more perfectly aligned teeth have fewer gum problems and teeth that can be cleaned more easily, which helps avoid dental decay. The benefits of orthodontic treatment can last a lifetime.

Now that you understand the importance of seeing your general dentist during orthodontic treatment, I'll share the story of a teenage patient. This patient was my son's friend from school. As is customary, after I referred her to an orthodontist, I continued to see her for routine checkups at 6-month intervals. She came in one day after school for a semiannual cleaning and examination. Upon examination I saw that her gums were inflamed and bleeding. It is always difficult to use floss properly around and underneath banded teeth that have orthodontic braces on them. So, I had my assistant help her to do it properly. Flossing correctly with braces can take ten to fifteen minutes daily. The patient must take more time to thread the floss, using a reusable plastic needle, to get under each and every wire between each tooth to remove the biofilm.

I told this patient that I wanted to see her again in two weeks' time because it would require that much time to stop the bleeding. When she returned, the condition had not improved at all. So, I called in the orthodontist, who was in the same building, to evaluate her condition. We both decided to remove the braces and allow her to floss more thoroughly and have her gum health return to normal as soon as possible. We spoke to the patient's mother, in person, to explain our decision. Her mother was adamantly insistent on keeping the braces in place. She wanted her daughter to complete her orthodontic treatment in the time that was promised. But we decided to stick with our plan, which had the patient's overall well-being prioritized.

My young patient was at the top of her class. I believe that the stress of maintaining straight A grades on her report card affected her gum health combined with the difficulty trying to floss under and around all of the braces. Once the gum health improved, the orthodontic treatment could finally be completed. Both the daughter and her mother were happy with the results and thanked us for our care.

The orthodontic staff usually teaches patients, both children and adults, to floss and improve or maintain their oral hygiene because it results in a long-term successful treatment. This anecdote emphasizes the importance of gum maintenance when undergoing orthodontic treatment with bands and braces.

Dental radiologist

One specialist whom many patients might not know about is the dental radiologist. Although all dentists have X-ray machines, the dental radiologist has two special X-ray machines that many dentists do not have: a cone beam X-Ray machine and a panoramic X-ray machine. These machines' X-rays provide more detailed views and reviewing them may be required. The cone beam machine shows hundreds of slices of the teeth and bony areas around the teeth. It is sometimes needed when the traditional full-mouth X-ray does not reveal specific areas adequately. The panoramic X-ray shows the entire jawbone of the upper and lower jaws, including the teeth. These additional types of X-rays are commonly needed for third-molar extractions, orthodontic treatments, and implants.

Oral pathologist

The oral pathologist is a dental specialist in diseases of soft tissues of the mouth and throat. Any biopsy from the oral tissues that a dentist or oral surgeon has obtained, due to suspicious lesions of the mouth, are reviewed by an oral pathologist. One of the lesser-known benefits of regular dental checkups is your general dentist is trained to do oral cancer screening. Unfortunately, oral cancer has a high mortality rate. The reason for this high mortality rate is that when a malignant tumor is found, it is usually in a late stage of development because the patient did not have routine periodic dental checkups.

I was told this fact by an oral surgeon, whom I had sent my patient to for a biopsy of a suspicious lesion on his throat. He called and told me that I had saved the patient's life. I remember the case well, as this patient was coming in every four months because he had heavy tartar deposits that needed removal to maintain better gum health. I always took the time to do a cancer screening and saw something that didn't look normal. After two to three weeks, when I asked him to return, it was still there, and I wanted the oral surgeon to do a biopsy. The oral pathologist reported that the lesion was cancerous. The patient had to have surgical removal, radiation, and chemotherapy, but he survived it all without any facial disfigurement or voice impairment. The early detection, biopsy, diagnosis, and treatment made the difference between life and death for this patient. This is why an oral pathologist is a valuable partner for most general dentists.

Dental anesthesiologist

Dental Anesthesiology is the specialty of managing pain, anxiety, and overall patient health during dental, oral, maxillofacial, and adjunctive surgical or diagnostic procedures. Hospital and office dental treatment for patients often requires a dental anesthesiologist because the patient cannot undergo certain routine dental procedures with local anesthetics. The patient might not be able to keep their mouth open due to some affliction, such as Parkinson's disease or another medical problem. This anesthesiologist is trained as a dentist first and can better anticipate the dentist's needs while operating.

I once had an elderly patient who, due to lack of periodic dental care for ten or more years, needed extensive dental care that normally would require more than eight to ten appointments of extractions, periodontal treatment, and prosthetic treatment for tooth replacement. I referred him to a hospital dentist because almost all of this treatment could be done in an extended hospital or office setting. The dental work needed would require general anesthesia by a dental anesthesiologist and procedures done by the hospital dentist, in three or four appointments. The extensive treatment this patient needed would not have been tolerable with only local anesthetics that general dentists are licensed to use.

Oral Medicine specialist

Oral Medicine is the specialty of dentistry responsible for the oral health care of medically complex patients. These specialists are also responsible for the diagnosis and management of medically related dental diseases, disorders, and conditions affecting the oral and maxillofacial area. The oral medicine specialist typically has extensive training in medicine and may also hold a medical degree. Several dental problems can be the first signs of more serious medical problems, such as Crohn's disease, halitosis, plumbism, bone loss of the jaw, atrial fibrillation, and leukemia. These diseases affect organs and soft tissues throughout the body but are sometimes first seen in the mouth or gum tissues because they can cause painful gum problems. While general dentists are perfectly capable of handling the usual dental issues patients present with, complex cases often go beyond the scope of a general dentist's expertise. Oral medicine dentists provide an invaluable service.

Orofacial pain specialist

Four years ago, the ADA recognized Orofacial Pain (OFP) as a specialty of dentistry. However, it is an unknown and unfamiliar specialty to many dentists and other health care providers. Since this specialty is so new, I have no personal experience referring to such specialists. However, I do have experience dealing with two conditions that OFP specialists might now be expected to manage. They are Bell's palsy and tic douloureux. Bell's palsy is facial paralysis due to lesion of the facial nerve resulting in characteristic distortion of the face. It is usually a temporary condition that disturbs the patient because it makes you look strange when you try to smile.

Facial pain afflictions, unrelated to the teeth, are not common. Tic douloureux (trigeminal neuralgia) causes extreme pain in the face from touching a trigger point on the face while talking, eating, brushing teeth, or even a gentle breeze on the face. It is a disturbance of the fifth cranial nerve which has a nerve branch that innervates the teeth, ears, and eyes. Most dentists only see this problem once or twice in a lifetime of practice because the people with this affliction are afraid of having a dental examination at which the dentist may touch their face and trigger the pain. Though these conditions may be uncommon, they can be difficult for the general dentist to treat. Especially if they have never read about or seen this condition. These rare conditions are why the new OFP specialists have recently entered the picture.

Public health dentists

Public health dentists are usually employed to oversee and conduct municipal, state, or national dental programs to promote oral health and prevent dental diseases within communities in underserved populations. These public health dentists are responsible for conducting oral health surveys and studies to assess the dental needs and trends within specific communities.

In San Francisco, there are five children's dental clinics that employ a public health dentist to organize and hire general dentists and dental hygienists. The dentists do treatment in an office setting, and the hygienists go to elementary schools to conduct dental health screening examinations. Parents can be directed to these city and federal subsidized clinics, if their child needs dental treatment and the parents do not have a dentist.

In summary, a general dentist can do a lot, and yet there are many recognized dental specialties for advanced dental needs. These specialists have deep knowledge and experience, and they sometimes work in specific facilities or with specialized equipment. Patients may go directly to a dental specialist for consultation or treatment. However, patients may be better received after being referred to a specialist by their general dentist. A referral can also be beneficial because the specialist may wish to consult with a patient's general dentist on the patient's behalf.

11

FOR DENTISTS ONLY

If you want to begin an in-office program to teach your patients how to use dental floss properly, this chapter is for you, doctor. The best way to start is to have a meeting with your staff and explain the importance of flossing to both dental and overall health. I posted an online video demonstrating how to floss for my students. Please visit https://youtube/9d51xUIlcTE?si=uNlkLLqSyamNVKZR to watch. Or just go to "Flossing Demonstration" on YouTube To get everyone onboard for this new service that you are going to offer your patients, it is mandatory that your entire staff realize that everyone can perform flossing better, easier, and more thoroughly than they may be doing presently.

After you have held that initial staff meeting, begin

by selecting a dental assistant or receptionist whom you want to teach this technique of proper flossing to first. You will train your assistant by having them learn by doing—beginning with their own practice of flossing.

Schedule twenty-five to thirty minutes of time each day for a full work week. It is possible that your first trainee may only require four days before they are able to floss all of their teeth to your satisfaction. At a time before the instruction week, prepare a periodontal charting appointment to record any bleeding areas. Promise your trainee that these new flossing efforts will stop any bleeding areas within ten days' time. This is just one of the goals and rewards of the effort to learn the technique properly.

Start each one of these appointments by using a disclosing tablet and with the staff member brushing in front of a mirror. Help your trainee to master flossing in front of a mirror, doing just the anterior teeth first. Then proceed to the posterior teeth. If your assistant can't do all of them correctly in the first twenty to twenty-five minutes, you can complete flossing the rest of their teeth. At the end of each appointment, record the progress. At the end of the week, ask your assistant to share with you their schedule for flossing at home on Saturday and Sunday. Record that commitment. Send your assistant home with a couple of disclosing tablets. Recommend flossing after dinner and rinsing and brushing before flossing. Schedule an appointment the following week for your assistant to demonstrate their flossing technique to you. Please always be supportive and complimentary on their progress.

Once you are satisfied that this assistant can teach flossing to another person, schedule them to train another one of your employees, under your supervision.

It is now time to work with patients. There are several ways you can get existing patients to volunteer for this program. Select a patient who always has bleeding gums during a prophylaxis. Or ask your hygienist to select such a patient who has this condition. Then you are ready to have this trained assistant to teach one of your existing patients. Call them up and bring them in for a consultation and explain what proper flossing can do to improve their gum health and how this can improve their general health. Tell your patient there will not be a charge as you are training your assistant who needs to practice her newly acquired skills.

Another way to initiate this program with your patients, once you have your entire staff trained and thoroughly flossing with a rock-solid daily habit, is to select a couple of your patients who have referred you the most patients. Call them up for a no-charge consultation visit and explain that you want to evaluate their home care personal hygiene. Do periodontal probing and see if they have two or three (or more) bleeding areas of their gums. If so, ask them if they would like to improve their oral health by scheduling a week of training at no charge. If they do, promise them that you can stop the bleeding within ten days. They will go home and tell their family and friends about what you did. Everyone knows of someone with bad breath that you can help because most halitosis comes from unhealthy gums and is reversible, in most cases, by better oral hygiene and/or gum treatment.

In case you have any concerns, know that "casting bread on the water" to help your existing patients by offering free dental services is ethically legal. Dentists do this all the time by charging less than their normal fees for loyal, longtime patients, especially those patients who may not be able to afford your current fee. Please note, though, if they have insurance, in some cases, this may not be legal. For instance, a co-payment that an insurance company wants you to charge your patient must always be charged for their listed services. However, most insurance companies do not list Oral Hygiene Instructions. So, for those patients, your charges for OHI are between you and your patient.

After you have consulted with an existing patient, you'll be more comfortable and at ease introducing your flossing program to the next new patient. It is always easier to recommend treatment to existing patients because you have an established relationship with them. With your next new patient who has two to three (or more) bleeding areas during the periodontal probing examination, offer this training to that patient before starting any treatment, not even a prophylaxis. Explain to the patient why regular prophylaxis (cleaning) does not solve the problem that they have. When discussion of fees arises, always explain to them that the insurance company, if they have insurance, will only pay for one appointment annually; and the insurance may not cover oral hygiene instruction appointments.

Because costs might be at the forefront of most patients' minds, it's important you be prepared to defend the importance of your flossing program to them. Just because dental insurance companies do not allow OHI, does not mean that the services you offer are not valid. You must often explain to the patient that insurance companies are in the business of making money for their shareholders. As the patient's advocate, you are responsible for improving their dental health, which can subsequently improve their overall health.

For new patients who are referred to you, introduce the idea that part of their treatment plan is to start with OHI. To make this statement, you must do a thorough "open examination." One in which the patient can see and hear what the findings are during your examination of the head-and-neck, oral cancer screening, each tooth examination and gum probing, X-ray findings (with intraoral pictures of the teeth, if possible). An assistant or a recording device documents this examination, ensuring that a written treatment plan can be provided to the patient at the next consultation visit.

During this initial examination, do not ask the patient if they floss their teeth. Give the patient twenty-eight to thirty inches of floss and ask them to demonstrate how they use it. If they need a mirror, be prepared to hold one up for them or let them stand in front of the mirror in your treatment room. Do not be judgmental, but you can ask how they learned how to floss. Most patients have not received instructions from a dental professional.

You should be able to describe what treatment is needed in a single-page letter plus the order of treatment priority. At the following appointment, give the patient this letter to read before you meet with your patient; ideally in a non-threatening room, not the operatory (treatment room). Be prepared to answer any questions the patient has. You should be able to relate the cost details and have a receptionist or office manager make the appointments and financial arrangements. I have found that patients do not want to discuss payment arrangements with the doctor. Patients are far more comfortable discussing money with a business manager or receptionist.

When you have presented your treatment plan letter to the patient, the patient can easily show a family member or friend, afterward, what you are going to do for the charges that were discussed, before any treatment is started. Oftentimes, the decision to go ahead with dental care may be a family matter that must be shared because of the costs. This letter represents a "best practices" way to start a trusting relationship with your patient.

What I have experienced in talking to patients about prevention of gum problems by teaching them to floss properly, is that not every patient is ready to go along with the program. Your patient may have other priorities in their life that are greater. They may not necessarily discuss these other pressing matters. But they came to you for treatment and cannot afford or may not have the time or cost to focus on prevention. If they are satisfied with only your treatment of their teeth and gums, they will return for checkups, and this will allow you to reevaluate their gum health. If your periodontal probing examination continues to show bleeding and pockets of 4 mm or greater in depth, you can offer them the prevention program again to improve their periodontal condition. Patients who learn to maintain healthy gums will likely refer others seeking preventive services.

By helping your patients achieve better dental health by their own efforts of daily oral hygiene home care, they will never go to another dentist. Partly because no other dentist took the time and concern to teach them how to become independently healthy. Moreover, you will have the gratification of knowing that you have made a significant difference in their general health for the rest of their life.

The next chapter will give detailed instructions of how to brush and floss properly.

12

HOW TO BRUSH AND FLOSS PROPERLY

Brushing and flossing are an essential part of your home hygiene. How important is flossing? Well, let me put it this way: If I could only take either a toothbrush or dental floss with me on a trip, I would select the floss rather than a toothbrush every time. Floss removes bacteria in the most critical places on your teeth. Besides, I can use a washcloth to clean my teeth when I do not have a toothbrush. Really, it works simply fine.

Begin enhancing your home hygiene by using disclosing tablets. The tablets can be purchased at most drug stores in the dental section. These tablets enable you to stain the materia alba (white matter) of your teeth that has the food stuff and bacteria stuck on to a reddish-pink color. These tablets show you what a toothbrush can remove. The stain helps you to see if you removed all of it. But to use the tablets correctly, it is important not to use any toothpaste; just water: That is because the toothpaste will discolor or not allow the stain to appear. Once you have perfectly removed all the stained areas, you will realize how long it takes to brush thoroughly.

Now let's take a closer look at when to brush.

Brushing

The best time to brush one's teeth is after breakfast and after dinner. It is also helpful to rinse your mouth first, with a cup of water, before brushing to remove some loose food particles. After lunch, rinsing your mouth or brushing again is recommended, for adequate oral hygiene as the object is to retire for sleeping with cleaned teeth and gums.

One reason for toothbrushing is to maintain a clean mouth during the day to avoid bad breath from digestion of food on the teeth. The other reason is to avoid having saliva that will become acidic, which promotes cavities. The third reason to brush teeth regularly, both day and night, is to avoid gum disease.

Most dentists recommend the following method for

brushing teeth: Place the brush at a 45-degree angle, pointing the bristles up at the gum line on the upper gums and teeth, then downward on the lower gums and teeth. The junction of the teeth and gums is where to place the brush. Then make a circular or vibrating motion, keeping the brush on the same teeth for three to four seconds before moving to another area. This method stimulates the gums and cleans the teeth adequately. You can brush back-and-forth on the tops and sides of your teeth, but do not brush back-and-forth along the gums. Two minutes of brushing twice daily is the ADA recommendation, which I also recommend.

Electric or battery operated toothbrushes can clean ones teeth in less time than manual toothbrushes. Another advantage that they have over manual toothbrushing is that the brush head is smaller and can reach around the last tooth in the arch more thoroughly. The other advantage is they are easier to use on the tongue side of the teeth. Personally, I prefer using the electric toothbrush, but I travel with a manual one as it takes up less space and it is still the choice for many folks .

Flossing

When is the best time to floss?

The best time to floss is before going to bed. At the end of the day, most people have more time for dental home care. As bacteria requires 24 to 36 hours to become an irritant to your gums, once a day or night is recommended. Besides, flossing requires more time than brushing. I used to recommend flossing in front of a mirror until you perfected the technique.

Why is flossing necessary?

Because the brush cannot completely remove all the biofilm between the teeth and in the cuff of gum space that surrounds each tooth. Flossing accomplishes two important goals for your dental routine. It removes food caught in the spaces between the teeth, and when done correctly, it removes the biofilm that leads to inflammation of the gums, a leading cause of many oral and overall health problems.

How to floss.

Regarding flossing, the first thing to review is how you are holding the floss. Don't grasp it with your thumbs and index fingers. In order to reach the back teeth, you need to use the tips of your index fingers and thumbs.

Flossing is easiest with short fingernails. Begin learning how to floss by flossing your front teeth first; the front teeth are much more accessible than your back teeth. When learning how to floss, practice in front of the bathroom mirror, so you can see what you are doing. Once you have mastered the front teeth, you will be more confident learning to floss the back teeth.

I recommend the Glide brand of floss, which is strong and not likely to break or shred. Those are the qualities to look for if you aren't able to buy Glide. Most other types of floss are too thick. (There are over a dozen different types of dental floss that are reviewed on YouTube. Personally, I use POH floss, but this brand is very thin and breaks easily if you are beginning to learn to use dental floss. So, stick with Glide when you first start out.)

I invite you to watch my flossing demonstration on YouTube after you finish reading this chapter. My video will help you to learn how to floss properly: It can be found by stating "flossing demonstration" or my name. I made the video for my dental students.

Please note: Later in this chapter I will cover some options for folks who, for any reason, are not able to use their hands or fingers to floss.

To begin flossing, wrap about twenty-eight to thirty inches of the floss lightly around your two middle fingers. These are your “anchor fingers.” Using your middle fingers as anchors frees up your thumbs and index fingers to be used to guide the floss. The ideal length of the floss between your guide fingers is one-and-a-half to two inches long. Most of the time, you will be using one finger near the center of your mouth and one finger or thumb between the teeth and the inside cheek. The back teeth require more distance between the guide fingers. as your progress to the front teeth, shorten the distance between the guide fingers.

After you have perfected the technique, wrap more floss on one middle finger than the other. As you floss from back teeth forward, unwind the floss from one anchor finger and wind the floss on to the other anchor finger. In this way, the floss stays cleaner.

Hold the floss at a 45-degree angle. Use a sawing motion to slip the floss between two teeth. Once there, pull back with both fingers to form a “C” and scrape the tooth three distinct times, moving your guide fingers in unison. Then pull forward and scrape the other side tooth three more times. Each time the floss forms a C shape by wrapping around the tooth. In total, you will be performing six up-and-down scraping motions for each interdental space. When flossing, make sure you include the sulcus (crevice) below the gum cuff. This is where the bacterial colonies can form. Repeat the sawing motion at a 45-degree angle to remove the floss from the in-between space; this is the best way to withdraw the floss.

Always start in the same place in your mouth to begin flossing, so you don't miss any teeth. I suggest you start on the upper-right canine, or cuspid (pointed tooth) and continue around to the other left cuspid tooth. Watch the video repeatedly as you practice nightly.

Another suggestion is to have your right hand outside of the mouth, and the left hand finger inside, when flossing on the right side. And, of course, you would have your left hand outside of the mouth and the right hand fingers inside the mouth when flossing on the left side. When you reach the midline of the arch, switch hands to correspond to the side you are flossing. You may need to watch the video several times to remember this flossing technique.

I recommend that you master doing the front teeth before trying to do the back teeth, as they are easier to do. Once you have mastered the skill of flossing the front and back teeth, try to teach it to a family member if you can.

My patients have asked me why so much floss length is necessary. Certainly, flossing can be done with a shorter length. However, using the longer length enables the user to change the floss from one anchor finger to the other, thus always working with a clean unused portion. This is a small matter because the same area of the floss used on all the teeth will disrupt the biofilm adequately. But using a new portion of the floss gives one a cleaner feeling knowing that each part of the floss is cleaner.

Without practice and training, dental flossing is hard to do properly. Dental supply companies understand this, and they sell many different types of substitutes for flossing. There are numerous types of devices, such as picks and small brushes, on the market. They are presented or marketed and advertised as tools that will help to remove food and bacteria, but this is malarkey—they might remove food, but they don't remove the sticky bacterial biofilm. It is the biofilm that causes the inflammation of the gums. These devices claim that they replace the need for using dental floss. Believe me, these claims are false and misleading.

As I stated before, the most crucial area needed for cleaning is below the gum and into the gum cuff, the crevice surrounding each tooth. Inflammation can occur here if bacteria is not disrupted or removed. This area is only accessible by dental floss and dental instruments used by dental professionals.

The other device that claims to clean the interdental area is the water pic. Water pics flush out loose food particles, but they leave behind the biofilm that sticks to the tooth and in the gum cuff. Unfortunately, using a pic gives folks a false sense of cleaning thoroughly. The water pic is available for purchase in some dental offices. Selling devices to patients for additional profit is inappropriate. Moreover, a water pic does not serve as a replacement for flossing.

If you feel you cannot master flossing from a spool of floss or you are now using these ready-made floss holders, please read on about my recommendation for their usage. There are devices available that have the floss strung or mounted on a plastic prong or fork. I have recommended these devices to some of my elderly patients who have arthritis in their hands. However, when using these implements, you need to do more than scrape up and down, once you have sawed through to gain entry between the teeth. You need to also turn the handle, this way and that way, while between the teeth, to try to encircle the tooth circumference and reach as much of the tooth as possible. In this manner, you can duplicate the C-shape wrapping and scraping of the sulcus below the gum and into the gum cuff.

Learning to floss properly takes practice over a period of time. Some folks may have better dexterity than others and can learn in just a few weeks. Others may require more time and practice. But the benefits are worth the time invested.

13

CONCLUSIONS, ADVICE AND THOUGHTS

The medical community now acknowledges the interrelationship between oral health and overall bodily health. As dentists we have always known this fact.

Inflammation of the gums and infected teeth creates a risk that toxic bacteria from the mouth can enter the blood and circulate throughout the body. The immune system becomes compromised and that can lead to disease and other negative health conditions. Poor dental health has been correlated with various serious conditions, including endocarditis, myocardial infarction, cerebrovascular incidents, diabetes mellitus, respiratory infections, pneumonia, oral and colorectal cancer, otitis media, Alzheimer's disease, and low birth weight in infants born to mothers with periodontitis. These diseases can stem from chronic gingivitis, which is preventable, or periodontitis, which is controllable.

The idea that the health of the mouth is important for overall health is not new. A notable discourse on the significance and value of teeth is discussed in Cervantes's esteemed novel *"Don Quixote: The Man of La Mancha,"* published in 1605. Don Quixote says the following to Sanchez, his sidekick: "I would rather lose my arm, providing it is not my sword arm, than lose a tooth. For a mouth without a molar, is like a mill without a stone, and a tooth is worth more than a diamond." Too bad Don Quixote did not say much to Sanchez about how he could prevent problems with his teeth and gums.

If you did not think flossing was necessary to maintain good oral health before you read this book, by now you realize its importance in preventing most problems of the teeth and gums. Moreover, you now know that the health of your gums has a significant effect on your general health and wellbeing.

In Dr. Michael Roizen's book *"Real Age: Are You as Young as You Can Be?,"* he states the following: "Flossing daily and seeing your dentist and hygienist every 6 months can make your Real Age 6.4 years younger." In fact, Dr. Roizen was invited to be a guest on Oprah Winfrey's TV show. She asked him what single health care practice can a person do to extend their longevity. Without any hesitation, Dr. Roizen said, "You should floss your teeth every night before going to bed."

Of course, you need to floss properly to prevent gum disease and to avoid the decay of an existing restoration. Finding a dentist or hygienist to teach you how to floss correctly remains a challenge, but it is a promising idea. Despite all the kinds of preventive procedures that are available, such as tooth sealants for children, fluoride gels, community water fluoridation, and silver diamine fluoride, you can still have a new cavity or decay of an existing restoration.

We have known for a long time that flossing and brushing is not enough to prevent cavities. What we put in our mouths—including what we should not eat too often, such as sweet things—can still cause cavities, despite all our good oral hygiene habits. Sugary foods and snacks are the main cause of dental decay.

A poor diet full of sweets can cause more than tooth damage, and it is worth learning about these additional health risks. A children's endocrinologist, Dr. Robert Lustig, who is on the medical school faculty at the University of California Medical Center in San Francisco, authored a book entitled *"Sugar: The Bitter Truth."* He specializes in helping obese children get back to normal weight and size. He maintains that sugar and high fructose corn syrup (HFCS) are the main causes of obesity, not eating fatty foods. Sugar and HFCS can be poisonous to our bodies when consumed in enormous quantities. Various forms of sugar are hidden in many of our drinks and foods. Because HFCS is cheaper and sweeter than sugar, food manufacturers are replacing sugar with HFCS in a whole host of packaged foods. Our bodies are ready to metabolize sugar, but they are not ready for fructose. Moreover, HFCS can cause problems that can lead to hypertension, inflammation, insulin resistance, and major disturbances of the pancreas. HFCS causes storage of fat by not allowing the hormone, leptin, to inform our brain that we have eaten enough food. Of course, Dr. Lustig also includes an obvious risk from consuming large amounts of these two ingredients to cause chronic dental decay.

Please pay attention to the food labels for HFCS and sugar. Consider reducing the number of juices in your diet. They contain too much sugar or

HFCS. I used to tell my patients that if God wanted us to drink juices, he would have created juice trees, not fruit trees. Bottled juices are a convenience food that neglect the healthy fiber contained in eating one piece of whole fruit.

You may not have any concerns about having a decayed tooth now. It is still a worthwhile idea to develop good prevention habits. Gums recede with age, exposing roots that are more prone to root decay due to lack of enamel protection. Upon aging, the space between our teeth becomes greater too with recession of the gum. It is harder to maintain healthy gums because there is more space between our teeth for food to lodge. Fortunately, we can have lifelong healthy gums, but for that, we do have to be more thorough in our home care and maintain periodic dental checkup visits.

The main criticism I have about present-day dental education is that schools have moved away from the basic teaching of prevention. Dental professionals need to learn how to floss to remove the biofilm that causes dental cavities and gum disease. And they need to teach their patients this vital skill. Removing the biofilm between the teeth and in the gingival cuff surrounding each tooth is more important to the health of the mouth than removing the food on the outer aspects of the teeth. Brushing alone is not sufficient to remove the biofilm.

Dental schools also need to teach students how to encourage patient home care and habits. Without an improvement in what a patient does at home, in their dietary and oral hygiene habits, the disease processes will persist. Additionally, I believe that a course on nutritional science should be in the curriculum. Dietary advice is necessary to control or avoid dental decay.

What I found in my years of teaching was resistance to changes in the school curriculum. This is a fact that is a reality from grammar schools to the ivy towered universities. Many times, new universities were established because of the resistance of existing universities and schools to change the curriculum. As I discussed in the chapter on dental education, dental schools started in the United States when the existing medical schools would not expand the dental curriculum. There needs to be more reporting back by the ADA's Commission of Dental Accreditation (CODA) to the schools and interested parties. The notices on dental curriculum changes from the profession by the CODA should happen more often than the current semiannual hearings. After all, the CODA is charged with determining what the dental schools should be teaching.

Finally, in all the years I have been reading our monthly ADA journal and the newspaper they used to publish, I cannot remember any reports by CODA of what new courses or proceedings the commission approved or recommended. As all dentists must stay abreast of new knowledge and continue education for licensure for the benefit of our patients, we should be made aware of what changes are occurring in the dental schools.

Using and having a dental insurance policy is complicated, to say the least. I would recommend that anyone who is covered by employer-provided dental insurance should ask their benefits manager what the coverage includes. If you have an indemnity type of policy, you can go to the dentist of your choice. This type of policy is the best dental insurance policy available.

After you retire, if the dental insurance policy terminates, you do not necessarily need to buy an individual dental policy. If you have had regular checkup visits and completed all the necessary treatment recommendations of your dentist, such as crowns and tooth replacements, you will be better off financially just paying out of pocket for your dental care. Purchase of an individual dental insurance policy is not a good deal for the patient.

On the other hand, if you have a recently acquired dental insurance policy, before going to one of the dentists nearby on a list of HMO network dentists, I recommend you go to the office of a dentist recommended by a friend. Get an explanation from that office of what your policy covers. If you like what you are offered and like who will be treating you, try them out.

If your new dental insurance is a PPO dental insurance plan, I recommend the same advice. Go to the office of your choice before making a treatment appointment. Find out what the policy covers and who will be treating you. If you like what you are offered and like who will be treating you, try them out. What I think is more important than the type of coverage of the dental insurance policy is finding a dentist whom you like and trust for a long-lasting relationship. This kind of personal relationship will more than pay for itself because the long-term patient will always stand out in your doctor's mind as a most valuable and deserving patient.

Community water fluoridation was intended to eventually reach a significant percentage of the public. CWF is not keeping up with the increasing population shift to the suburbs and rural areas. It was always known that CWF would not reach everyone, but now we see that after seventy-nine years, only 63 percent of the public is receiving the benefits of CWF nationally. Worse yet, in California, only 58 percent of the public has access to CWF.

Moreover, some communities are dropping CWF, as costs are greater than when they initially started. The rising cost of maintenance is a factor in discontinuation of CWF. If the ADA and its affiliate state organizations genuinely believe that fluoridation is a way to improve the dental health of the public, it should allow the usage of salt fluoridation, as an addition to CWF. Because salt fluoridation has a proven record and everyone uses table salt in food preparation, it should be an easy decision to promote fluoridated table salt to reach the people whom CWF cannot reach. Just as you do not need to drink more fluoridated water to have the benefits of fluoride, you do not need to eat more fluoridated salt to have the required amount of fluoride to have its benefit of less cavities.

The ADA should be able to articulate the need for the continued usage of CWF where it is available and salt fluoridation where CWF is not available. Both kinds of fluoridation are necessary to end the disparity of dental health due to where children live. After all, the ADA claims to be the guardians of the public's dental health. Has the ADA become so bureaucratic and top heavy that they have lost sight of the forest through the trees?

The American public has access to a wide variety of consumer goods, ranging from automobiles to toothpaste. They should be able to make a healthy choice for their children. It must start with the profession that started CWF in the interest of improving the dental health of the public. It is up to the ADA, CDC, USPH, FDA and other dental health care organizations to take a leadership role and offer the public a healthy choice. If they do not pursue improving the dental health of children and young adults by allowing the availability of fluoridated table salt in the U.S., I believe that an informed public will.

The folks who feel they cannot afford the services of a private dentist have a safety net of subsidized dental clinics that are available in cities and towns for Medicaid patients and for patients who have HMO and PPO dental insurance plans. Subsidized clinics serve lower-income patients but have specific limitations on the types of services they provide. But they are still subject to a dental insurance's policy of allowed procedures and fees.

These clinics are also treatment-oriented and do not teach prevention to control the diseases that brought the patient to the clinic. If oral hygiene instructions are among the list of allowed procedures, no more than one visit per year is allowed. And, as I have explained, it is just not possible for a patient to learn proper dental care in one or two visits per year.

Moreover, subsidized dental clinics are less likely to offer the continuity of dental care with the same dentist over an extended period. Although some of the dentists will remain for an extended time, most will move on to more challenging private practices that can also be more financially rewarding. This fact makes it harder for patients to build a long-term relationship with their dentist, which is essential for the best quality care and for learning how to prevent tooth and gum diseases.

If you are going to one of these subsidized clinics and you like the dentist who is treating you, this is my advice: Ask the dentist to let you know when they may be leaving to set up a private dental practice. In this way you can continue with this dentist's care and benefit from your patient loyalty. Believe me, doctors appreciate a patient's loyalty.

Unfortunately, because they do not teach prevention for control of dental diseases, these clinics become like revolving doors. Patients return because their oral hygiene and dietary habits have not improved, so they come back with recurrent dental problems that could have been prevented.

Besides the presence of subsidized dental clinics for lower-cost dental care, dental corporations have come into being that provide another place for dental services. However, I am wary of dental corporations employing dentists for a profit motive with no state-regulatory oversight. Dentists are granted licensure by their respective states, permitting them to provide dental care to the public in accordance with established rules and regulations. For instance, dentists must always place patients' interests ahead of their own interests. The state requirements for corporations are not as stringent nor do they meet the standards of a health professional's obligations to the public.

What is needed is legislation to monitor and regulate these dental corporations for the protection of patients and for the avoidance of fraudulent business practices. The regulations should require dental corporations be periodically inspected for fair business practices to avoid illegal business dealings.

Notable physicians and public health doctors are on board the flossing wagon, reiterating the importance of flossing to your general health and longevity. Harvard Medical School's newsletter includes flossing as one of the five most important things to do for your health. Dr. Peter Attia, MD, author of the book "*Outlive: The Science and Art of Longevity,*" recommends regular dental visits and the importance of flossing.

Flossing is extremely important. The health of your teeth and gums requires daily disruption or removal of the biofilm between the teeth and the crevice between the teeth and the cuff of gum encircling each tooth. Dental researchers say it takes the biofilm 24 to 48 hours to grow and colonize the bacteria to cause inflammation. So, it may not be mandatory to do this flossing daily. Still, I recommend that you practice the daily habit of flossing each evening as well as brushing twice a day, after breakfast and dinner. As our immune system weakens from our youthful years to old age, gum tissues need an almost immaculate clean condition to stay healthy.

Of course, keeping our teeth healthy depends on more than just the removal of biofilm. We should limit or restrict consumption of sugary, processed foods. Dental decay can occur at any age. So many of the foods we buy in a package or cereal box contain more sugar than we should have in a healthy diet. And that goes for the sake of our waistlines too. Please ensure that you read the label to determine the sugar content and caloric value of the product you are purchasing. The best advice I once read about this is not to go to the supermarket hungry. Because if you do, it will influence your choice of selecting snack foods that are generally higher in sugar and calories.

Psychologists agree that establishing a good habit or change in behavior can take six to eight weeks. Just as unhealthy habits take time to stop, good habits take effort and time to adopt and keep. Much of the information from my experiences with thousands of patients has been presented in this book. Now you know what I spent my lifetime helping my patients to know. This knowledge that you have acquired is only of value if you can improve your dietary habits and oral hygiene habits. What you do in caring for your teeth and what you choose to put in your mouth every day will make a significant difference in improving and maintaining, not just your dental health, but your general health lifelong.

ACKNOWLEDGMENTS

The people listed below are dentist and hygienist friends I interviewed for an article I was writing. I developed that writing into this book. I am also thanking dental friends who unknowingly helped me.

Bob Barkley, George Gillespie, Joseph Zingale, Tom Kuhn, Bill Tognotti, Craig Yarborough, Mark Topoozian, Kim Benton, Larry Radcliffe, Rosemond and Arthur Muncheryan, Bill Sands, Liza Karamardian, Norman Chun, Mary Swift, Johnny Johnson, Steven Chan, Barry Kaylor, Tigran Avetisyan, Helen Yu, Ariane Terlet, David Rothman, Martha and Don Missirlian, Rafi Balabanian, Michael Parrett, Carolin Baghoomian, Martin Chin, Lauren Chin, David Refaee, Nick Ohanian, Raisa Galustyan, Donald Ruddell, Lowell Davis, Bill Tennant, Aparna Aghi, Howard Pollick, Richard Craeghe, Rick Leeds, Gary Kevorkian, Jana Kaye, Nishan Odabashian, Armand Bedrossian, Edmond Bedrossian, Bill Van Dyke, Gary Arabatyan, Norman Plotkin, Debra

Finney, Tim Baker, John Boghossian, Dennis Song, David Brown, Andre Dervi, and Steven Kezian.

I want to thank my students and patients who inspired me to author this book. My dentist, mentor, and senior associate dentist, Dr. T. Galt Atwood. His care, guidance, and friendship helped me through a challenging four-year dental education.

I must also thank my sister Antica Odabashian who introduced her employer to me and of course, thanks to all my family, especially my wife, Marie. They provided the necessary support and motivation for me to complete nine years of college and to contribute to improving dental health. Special thanks to my nephews, Jeffrey Ovian and Wayne Saroyan, for their comments on the manuscript.

I hope this book helps my students to be the fully engaged dental professionals that they can be with an ability to place their patient's interests ahead of their own. I wish them to experience the gratification of knowing that one's care can change a patient's life for the healthier and for the better.

I also owe my thanks to my editors, Matthew Ross and Jennifer Pellman, for their assistance, encouragement and advice.

A major portion of this book's profits will go to the Armenian General Benevolent Union in New York City for the implementation of Salt Fluoridation in the Republic of Armenia to benefit the children and young adults' dental and medical health.